What Happens When Someone

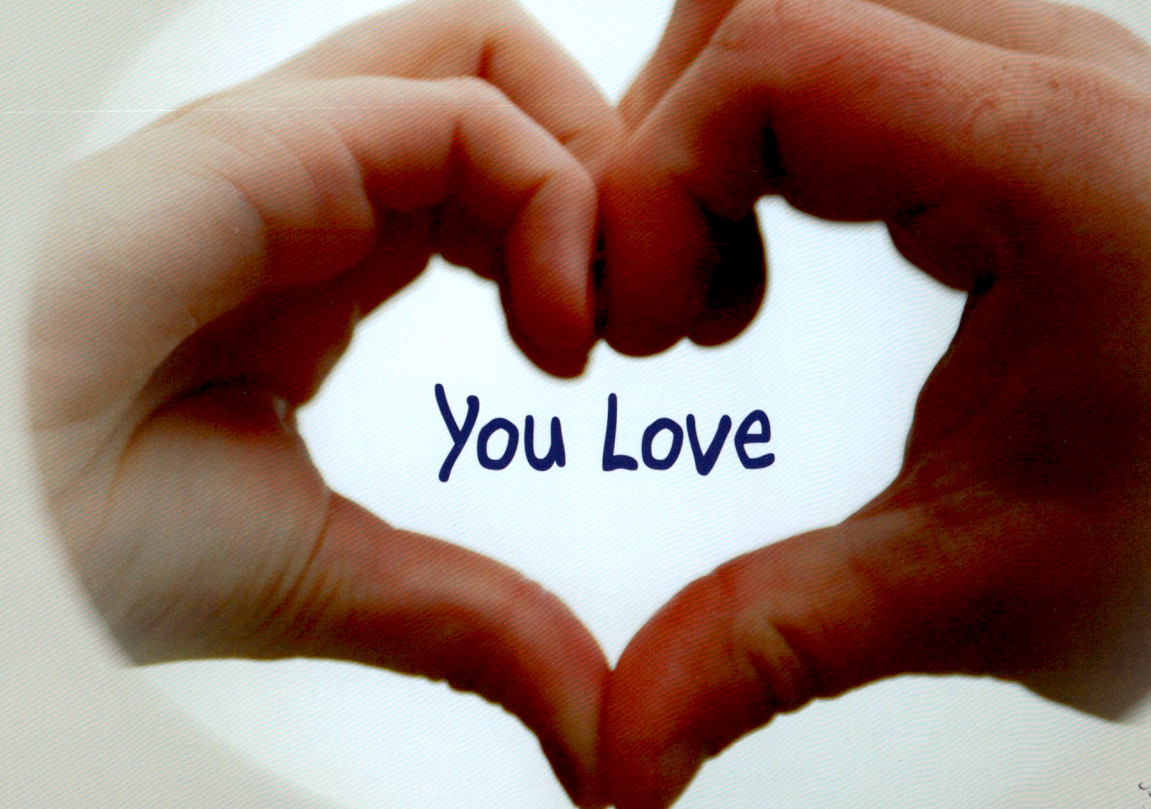

You Love

Has Cancer?

By Tonya Caudle

What Happens When Someone You Love Has Cancer?

Copyright® 2010 by Tonya Caudle

All rights reserved. No part of this book may be reproduced or transmitted in any form or by any means, electronic or mechanical including photocopying, recording, or by any information storage and retrieval system without permission in writing from the copyright owner.

Published by Caudle Creations
North Carolina

ISBN 9780-615-37680-6
Library of Congress Cataloging-in-Publication Data
This book was proudly printed the the United States of America
by Arrowhead Printing, Greensboro, NC

Author: Tonya Caudle
Photographs: Tonya Caudle

Contact: WhensomeoneYouLoveHasCancer@yahoo.com

This book is dedicated to

my children Timmy, Destiny, Brianna, and Tanner

and my husband Phil.

Also to all the families who suffer

from this tragic disease.

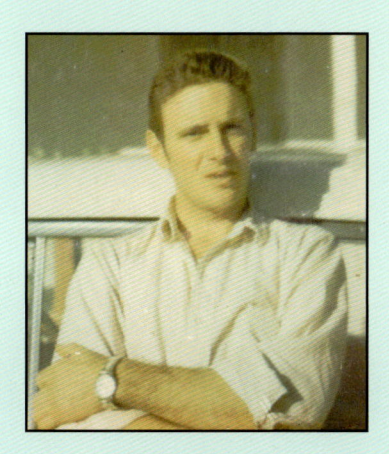

In Memory Of:
My Daddy
Thomas Hayston Ferguson

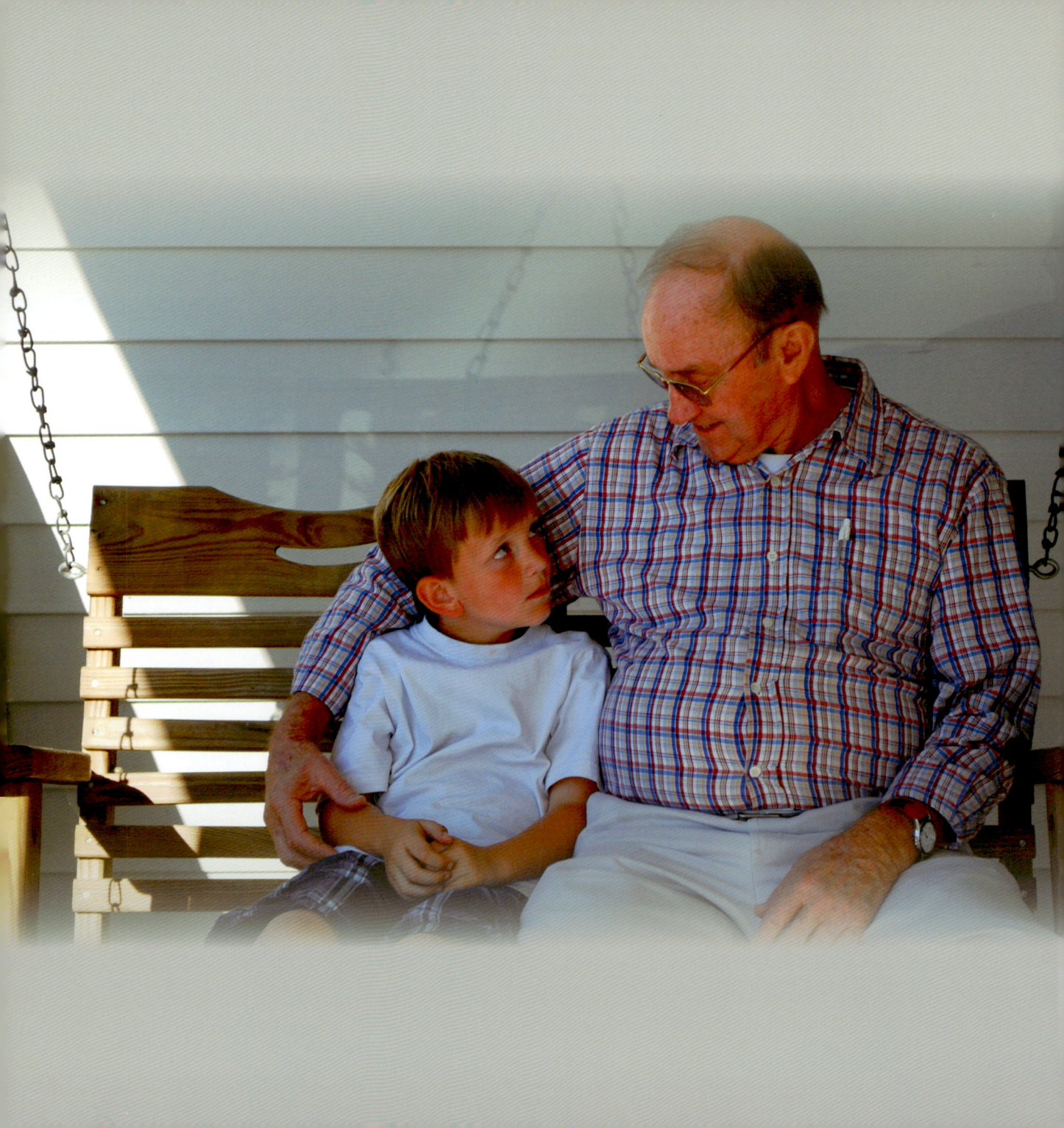

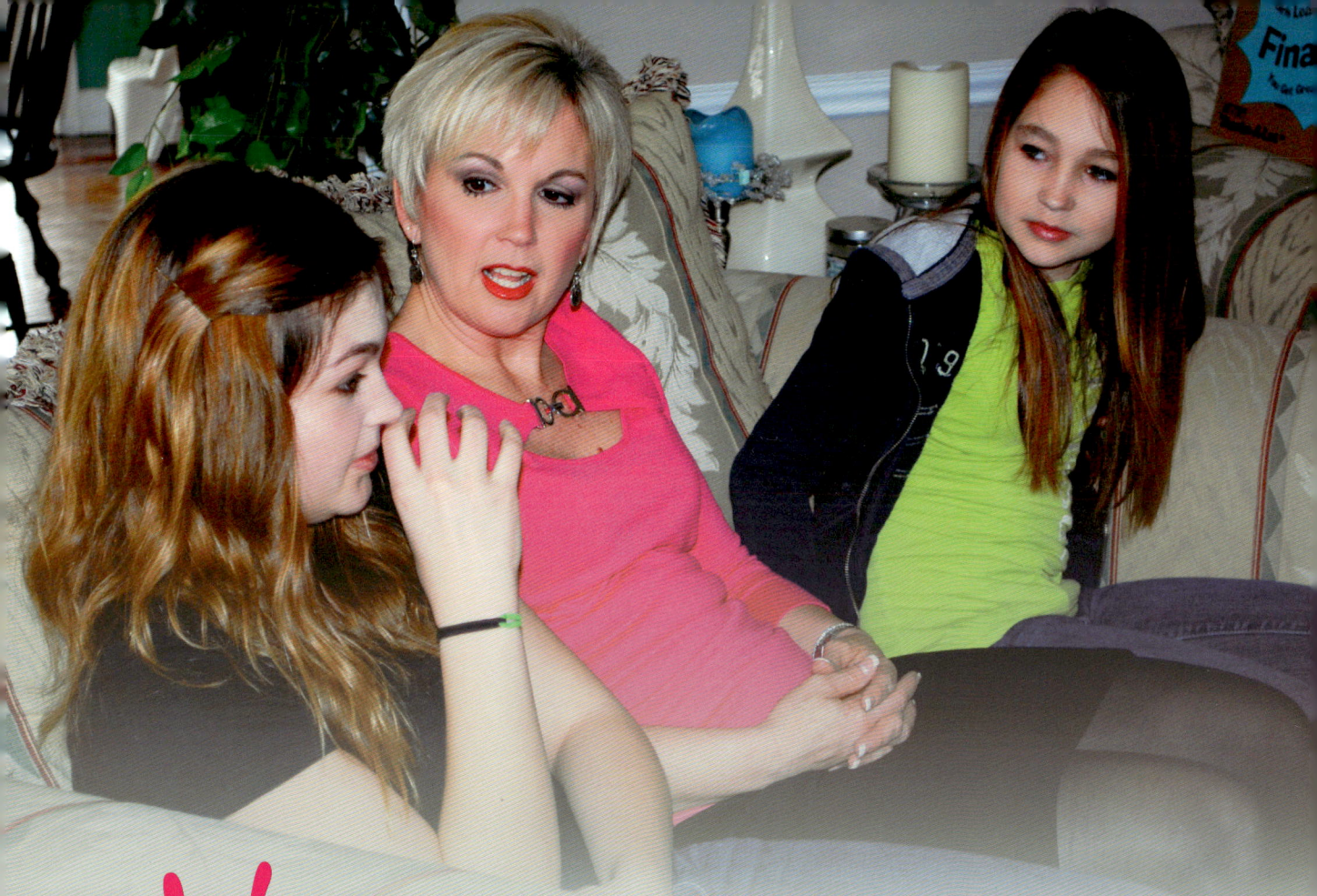

When someone you love finds out they have cancer, you feel sad and worried.

You don't know what to expect . . .

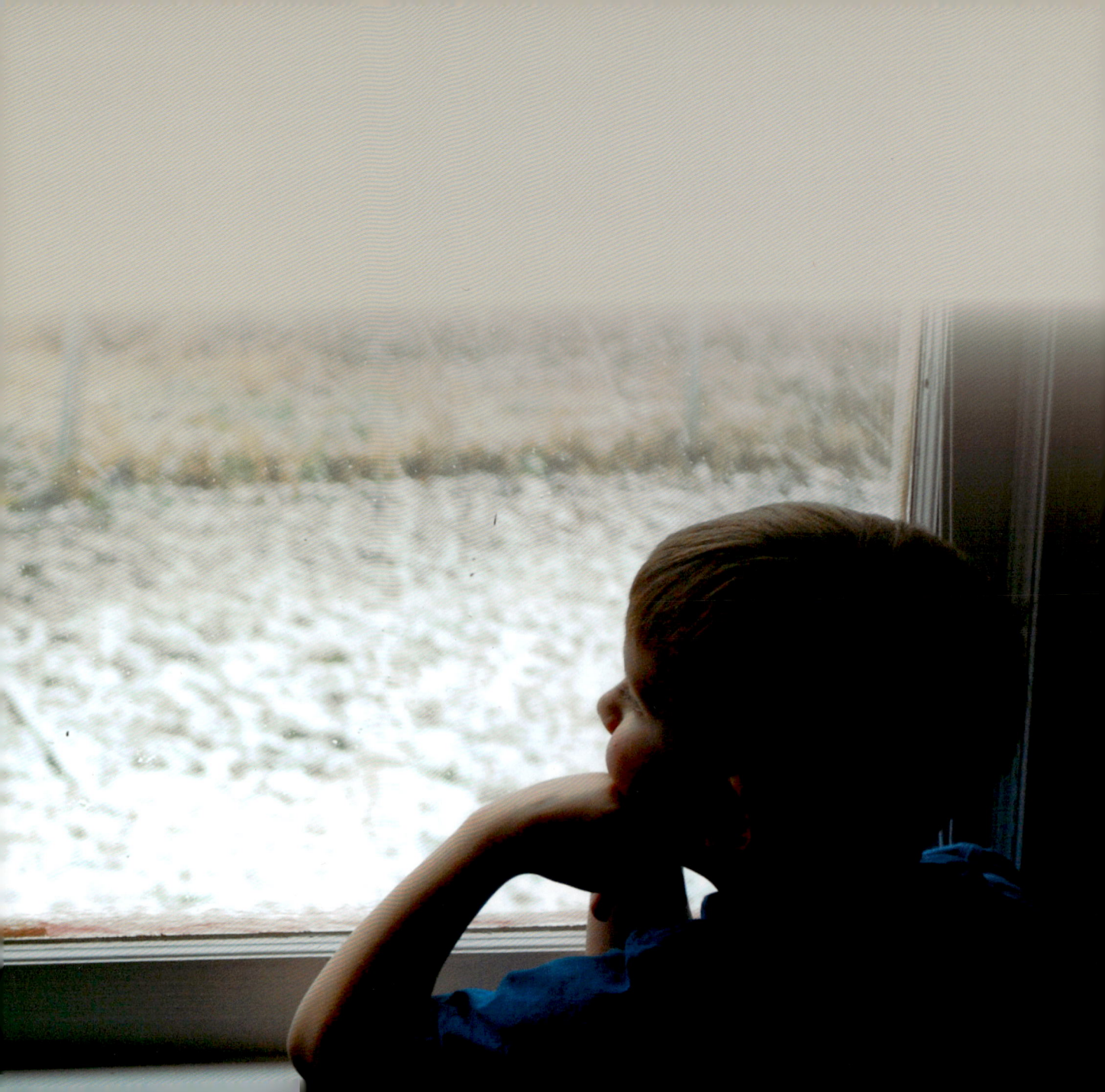

Cancers are bad cells in the body that make you

sick!

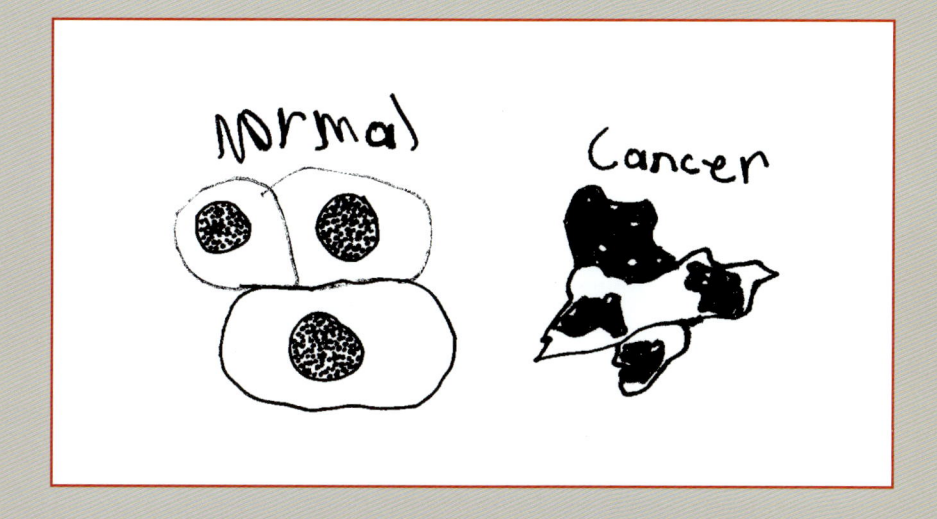

Normal   Cancer

10046

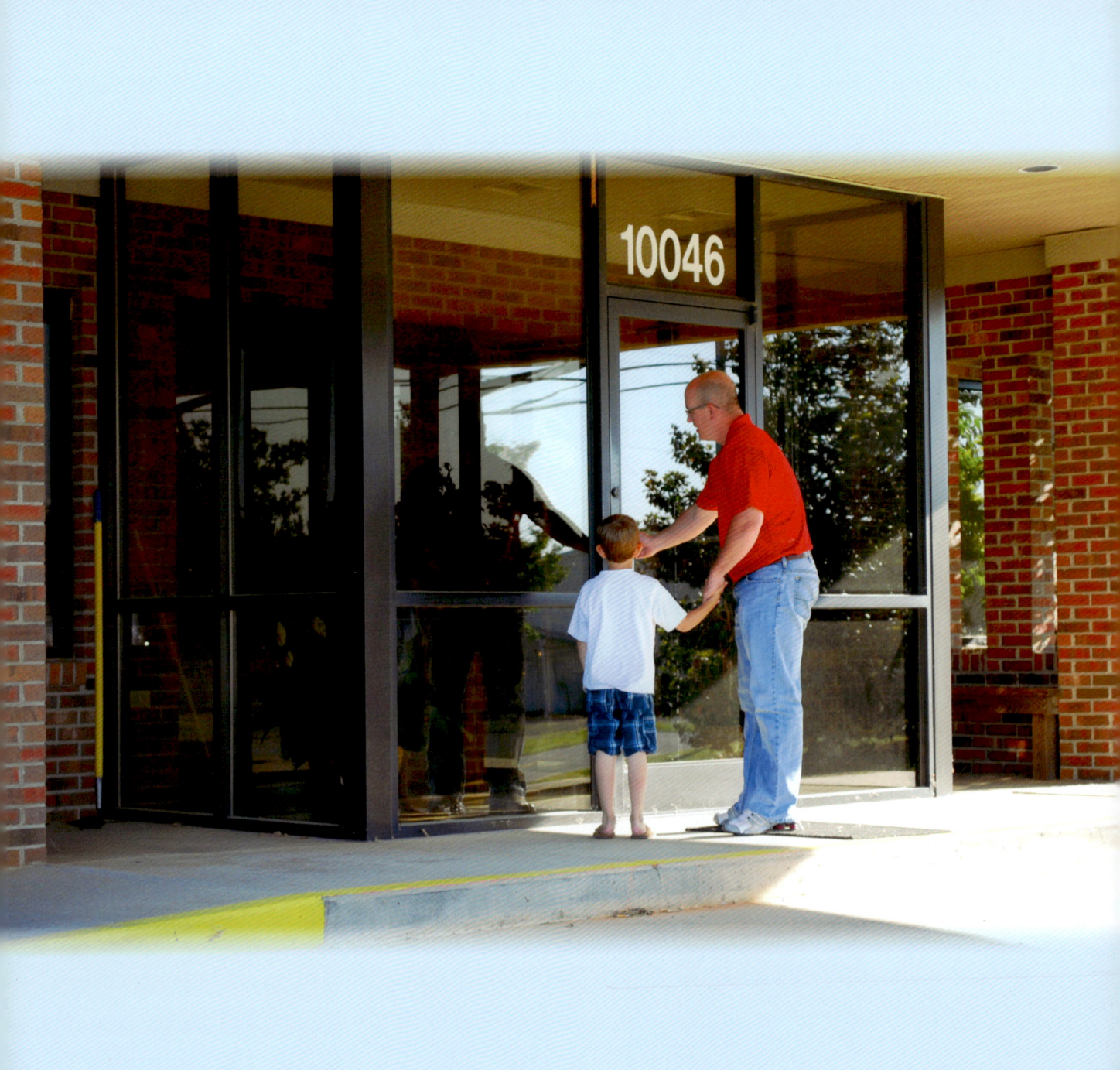

When they have cancer, they will need to go to the doctor for a lot of **check-ups.**

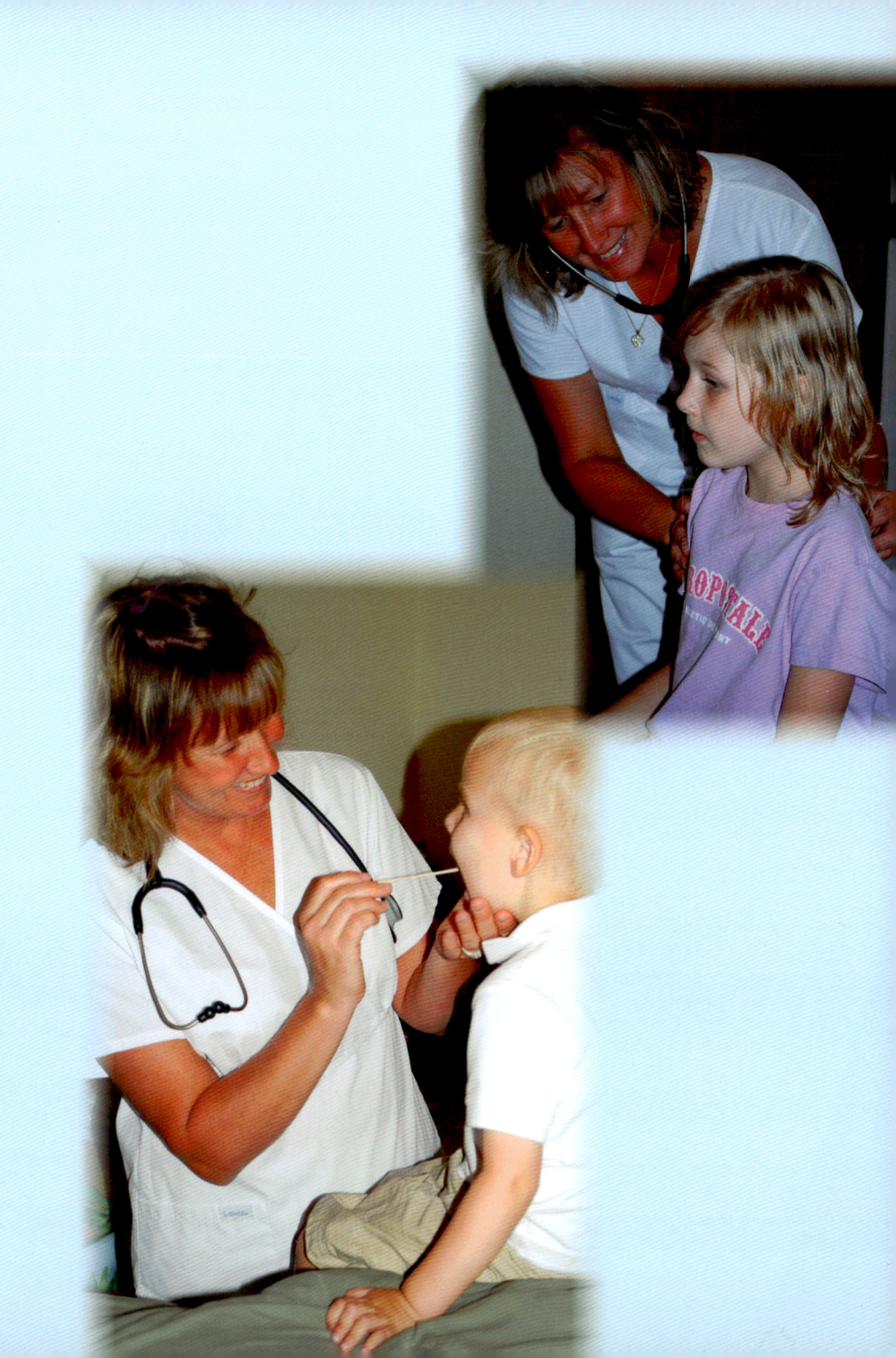

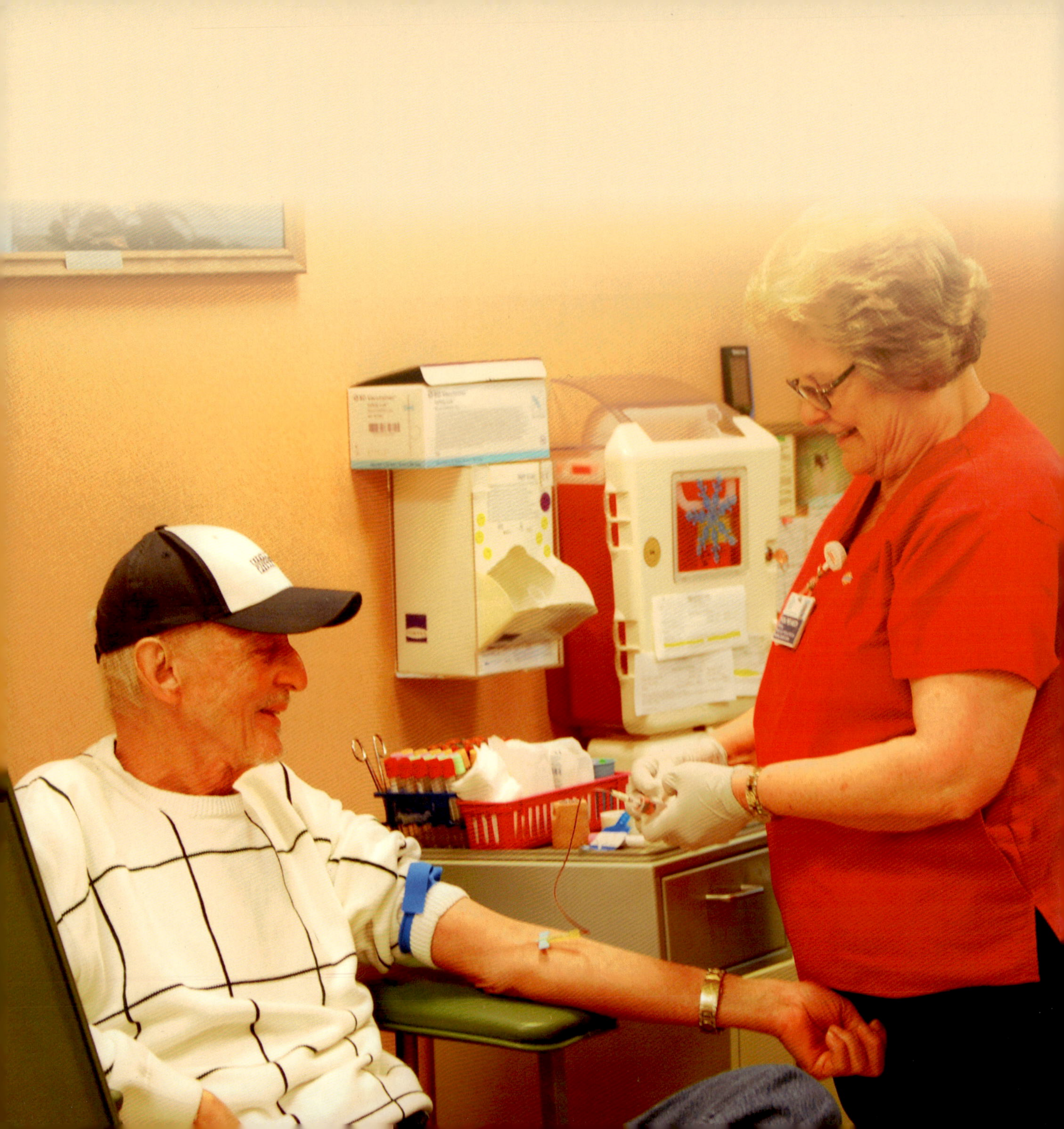

They will need to have blood drawn a lot to be

tested . . .

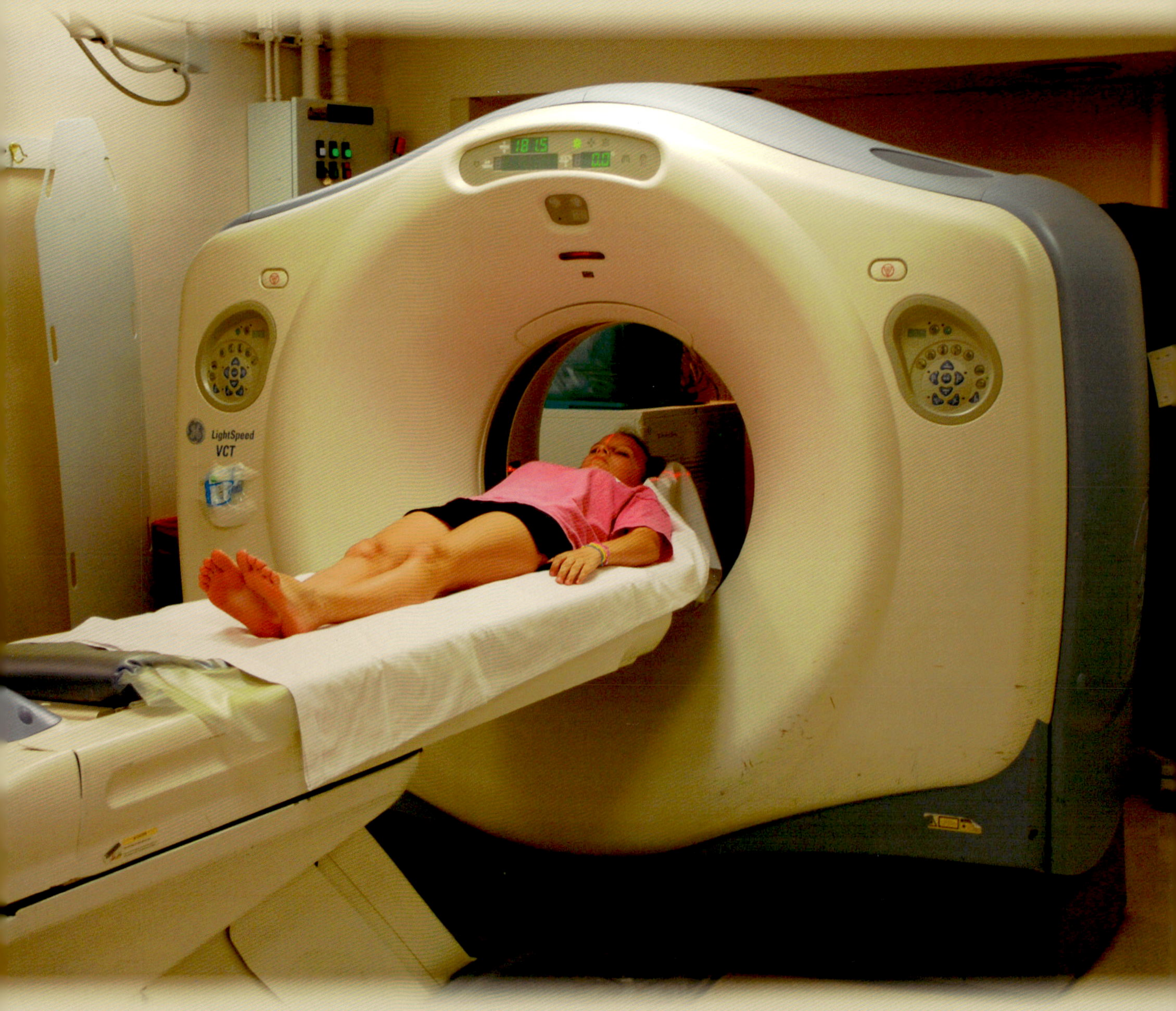
LightSpeed
VCT

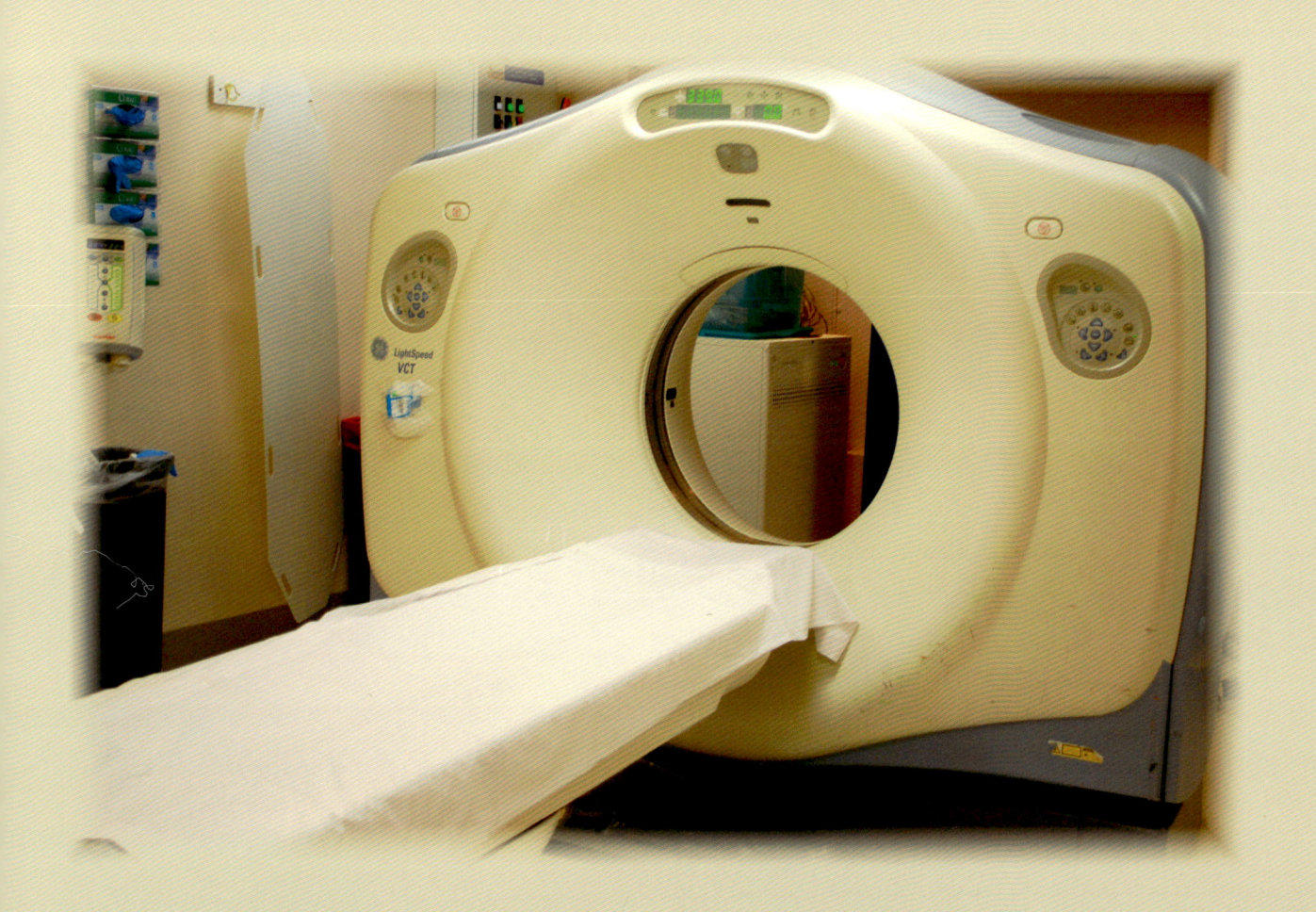

The doctor may send them to get a

scan . . .

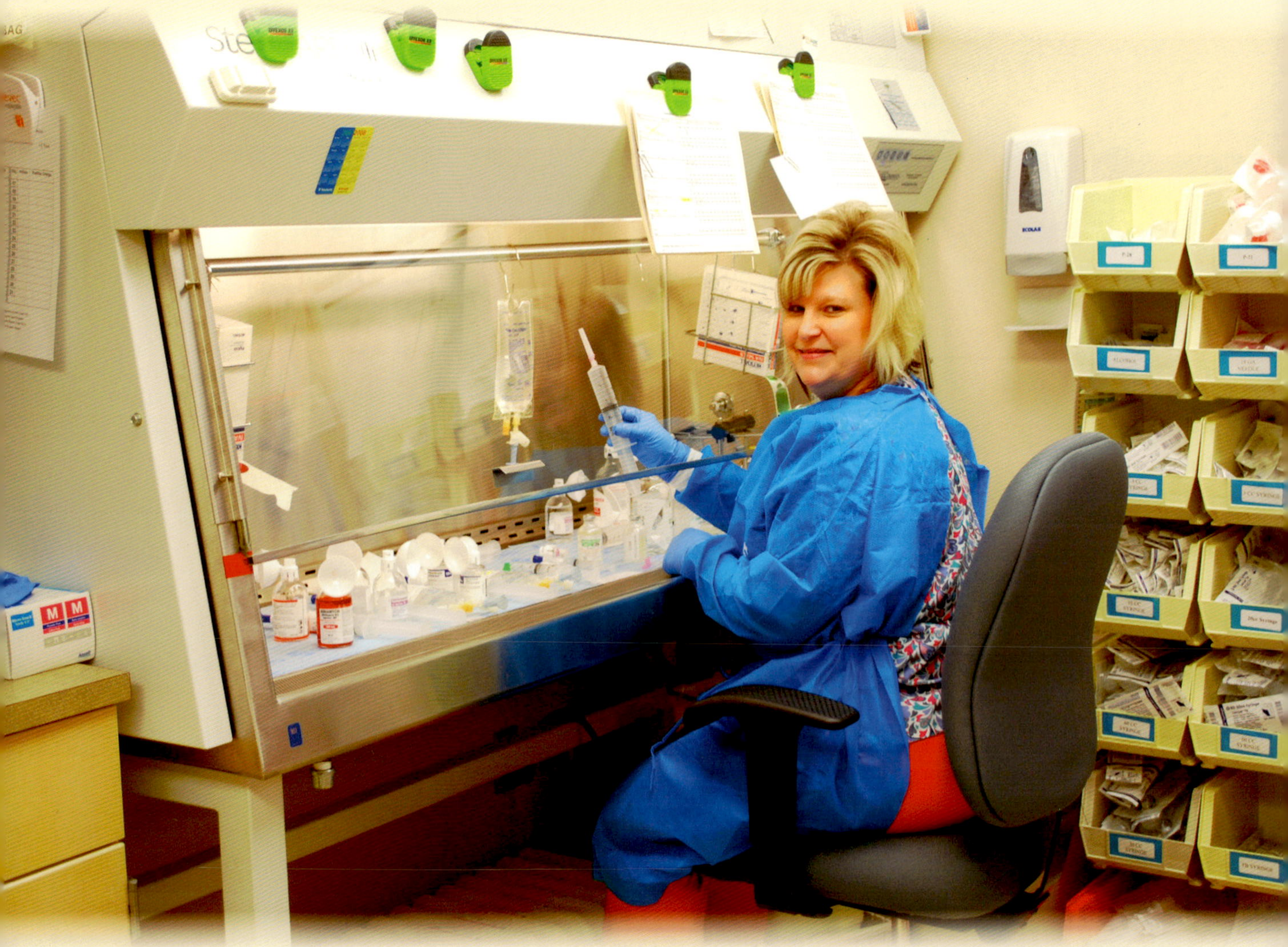

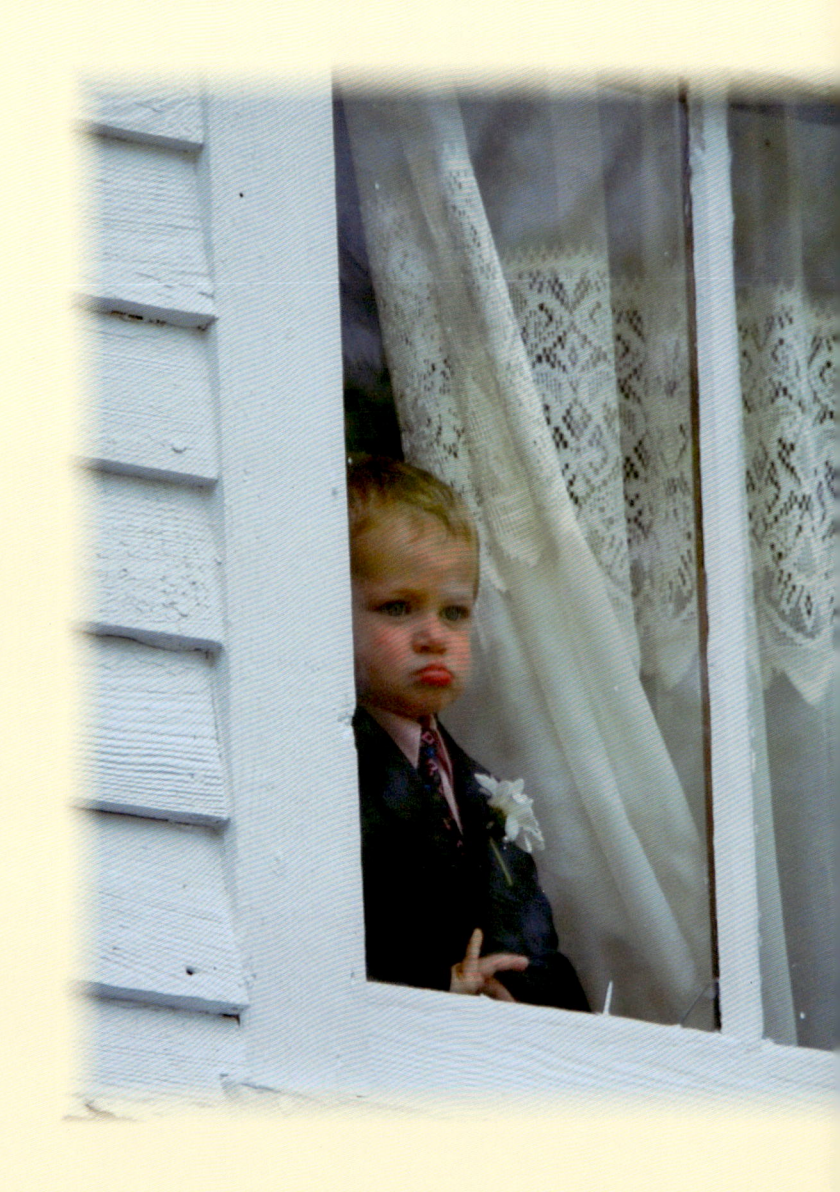

This will let the doctor know **where** the cancer is.

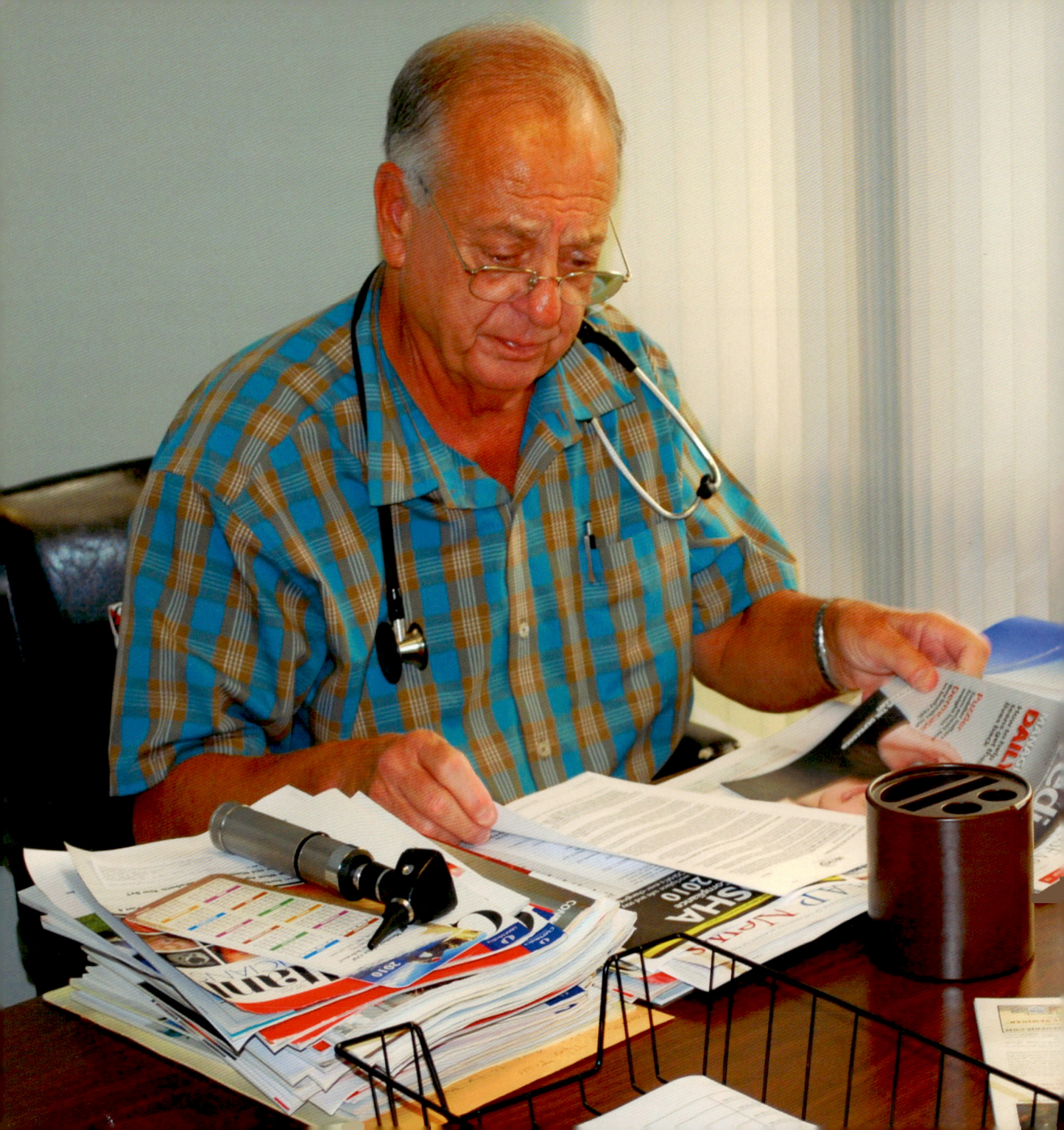

When the doctor knows where the cancer is, he will know how to **treat** it.

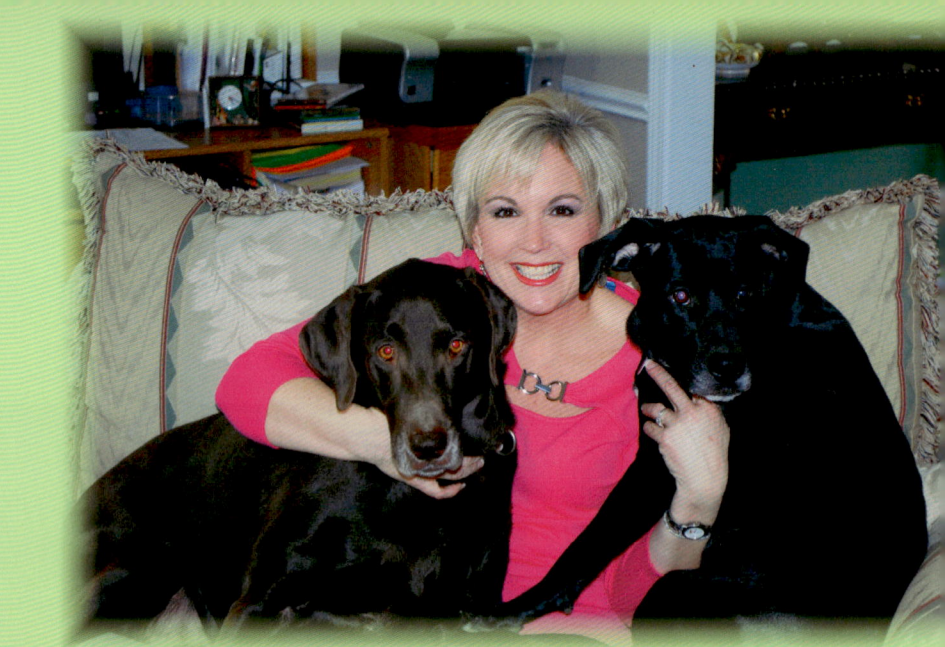

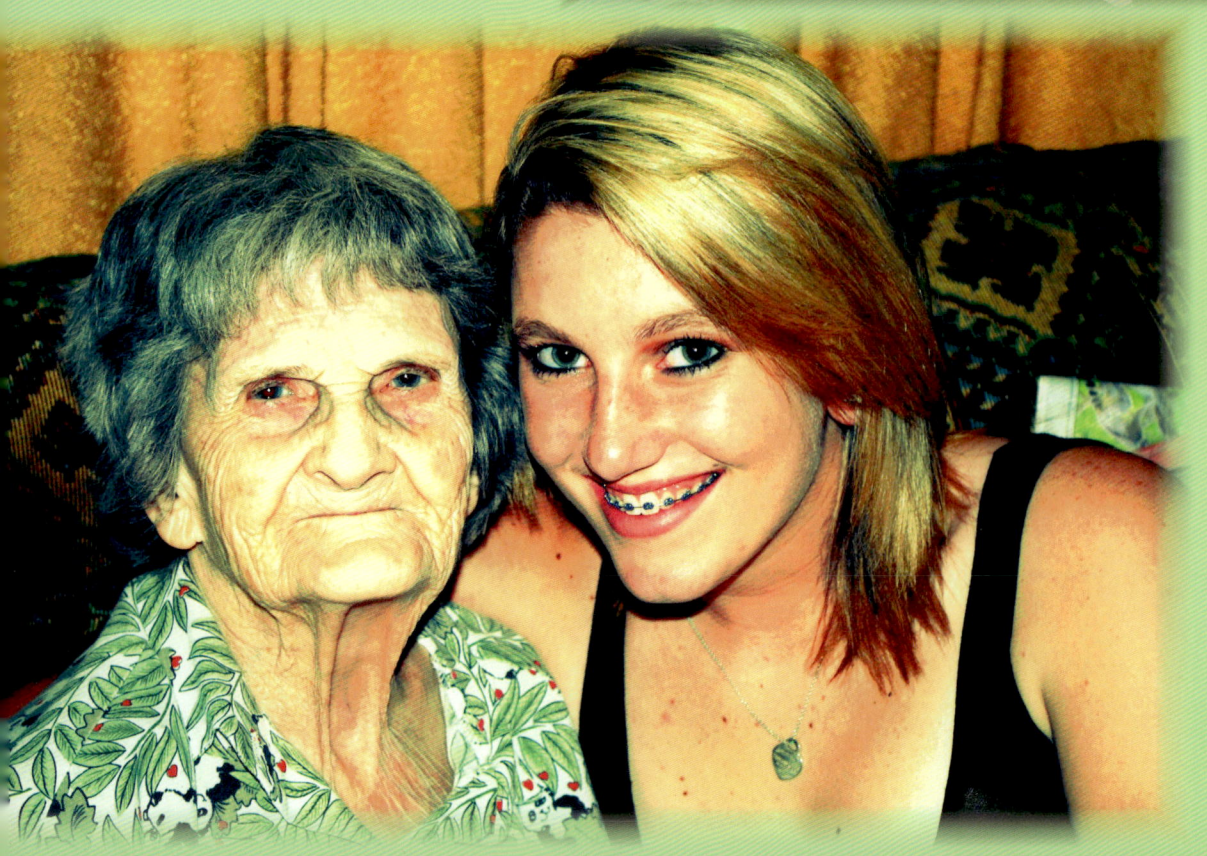

The doctor will then try to make them feel *better*.

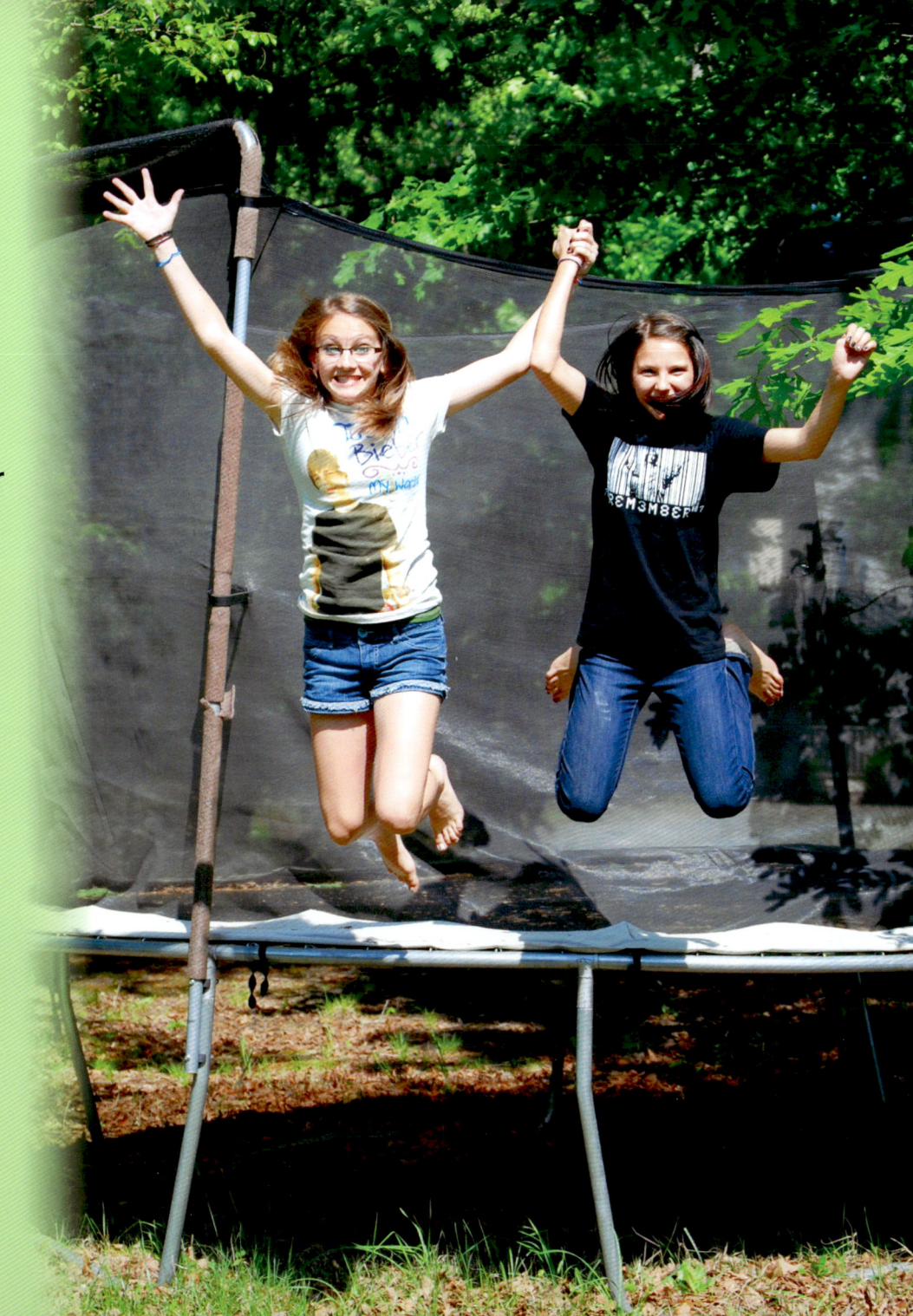

← CT/MRI/NUC. MED
← X-RAY

The doctor may want them to have radiation.

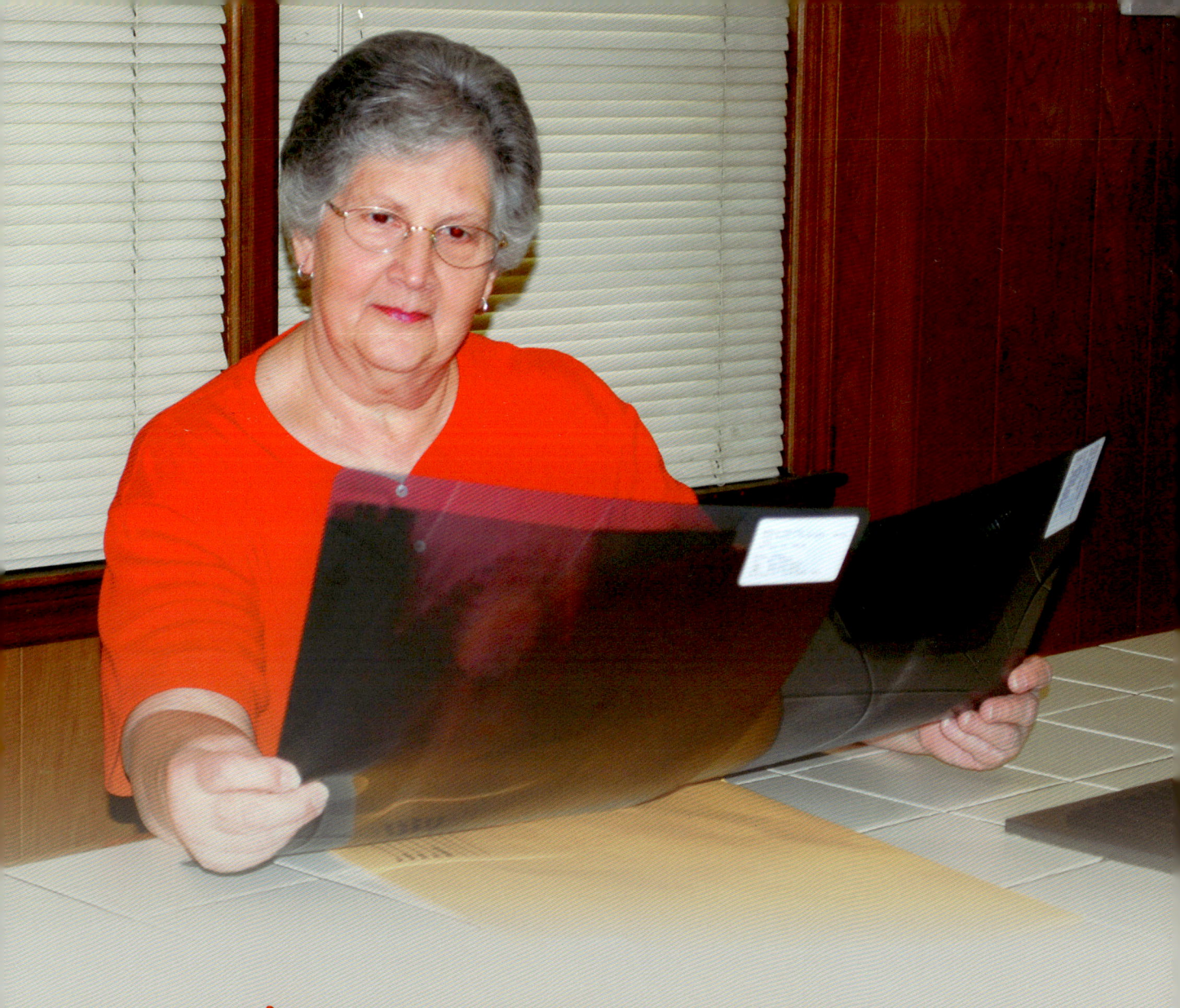

Radiation is like taking an X-ray.

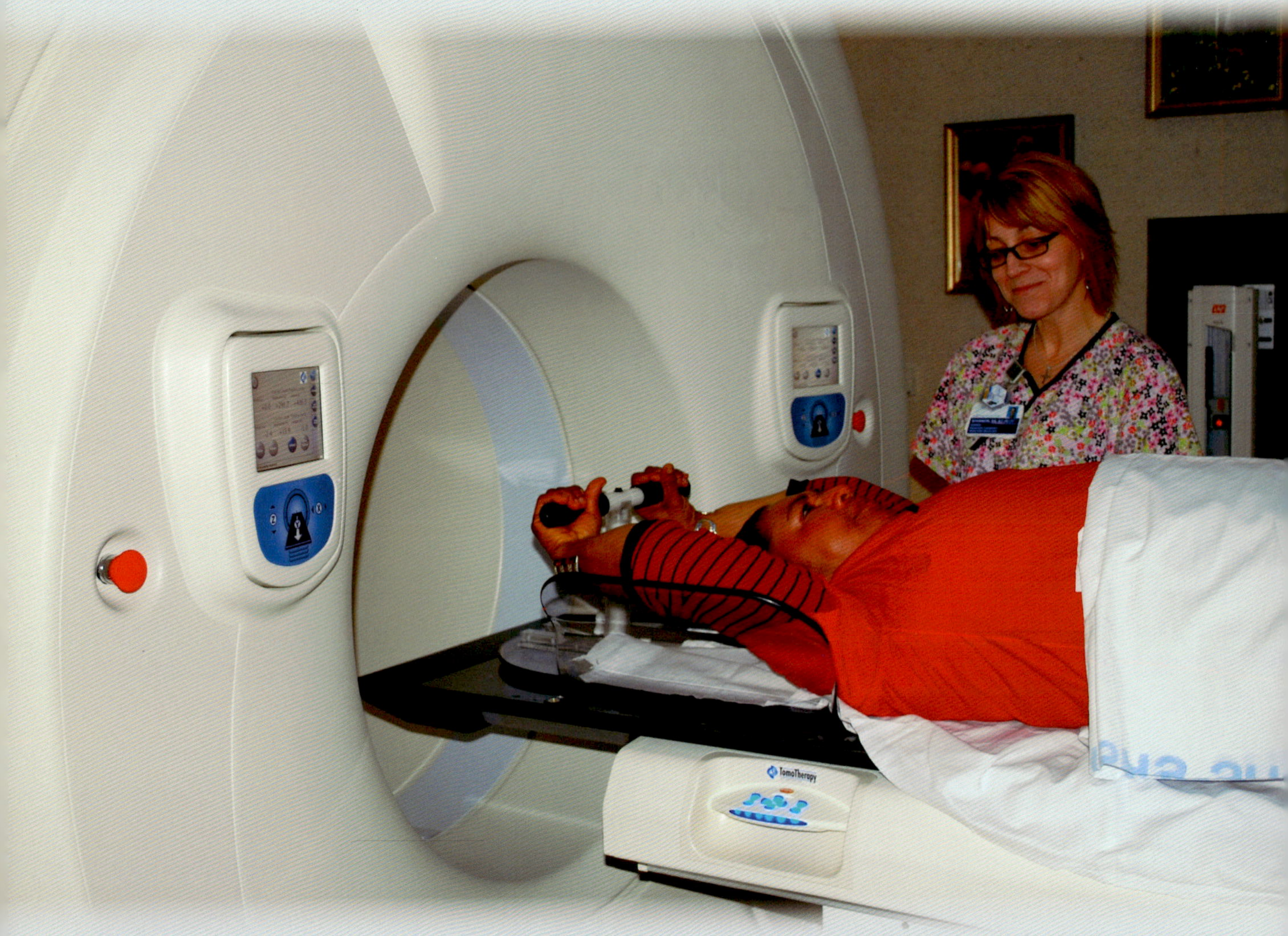
TomoTherapy

It zaps the cancer and tries to make it go away.

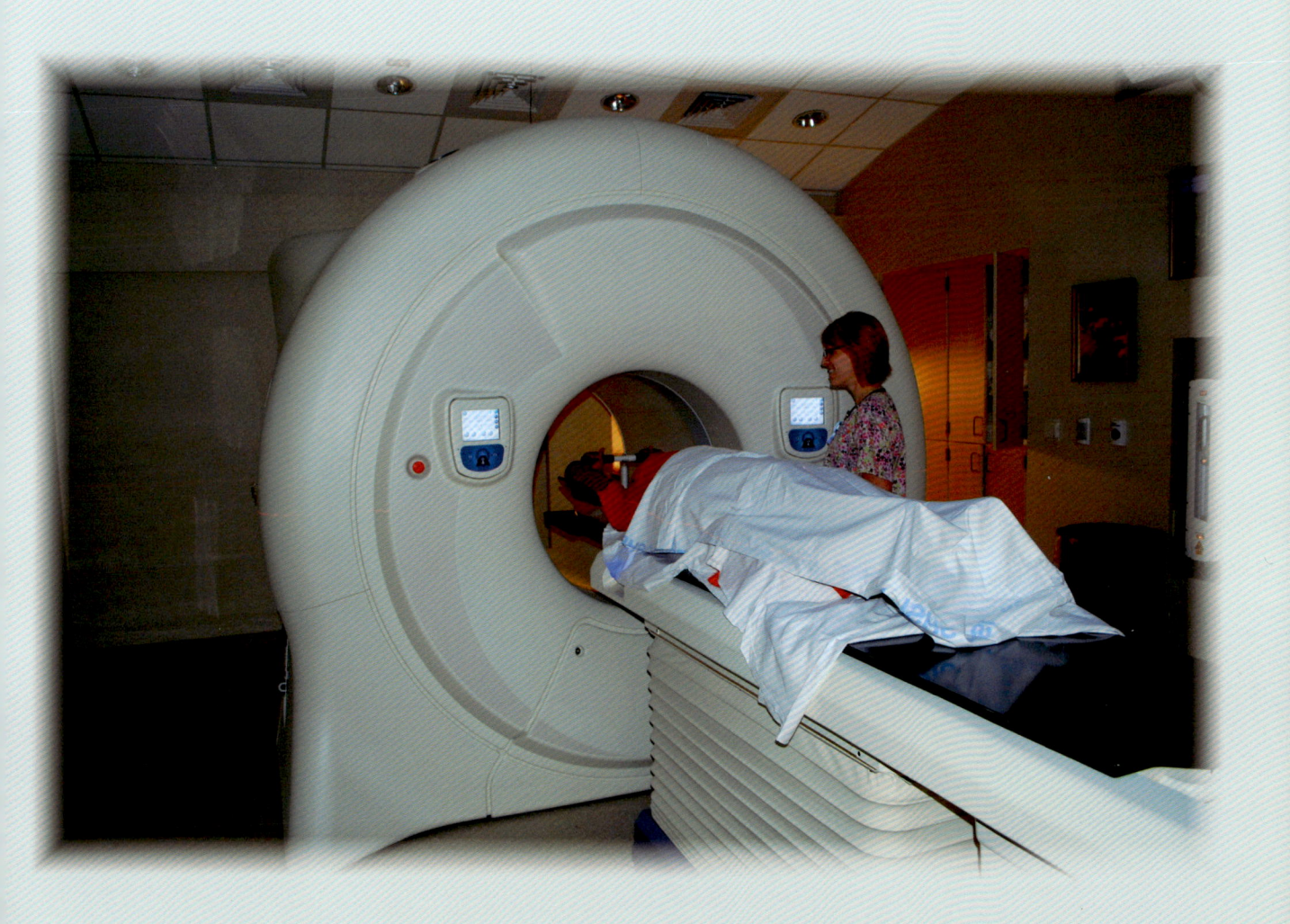

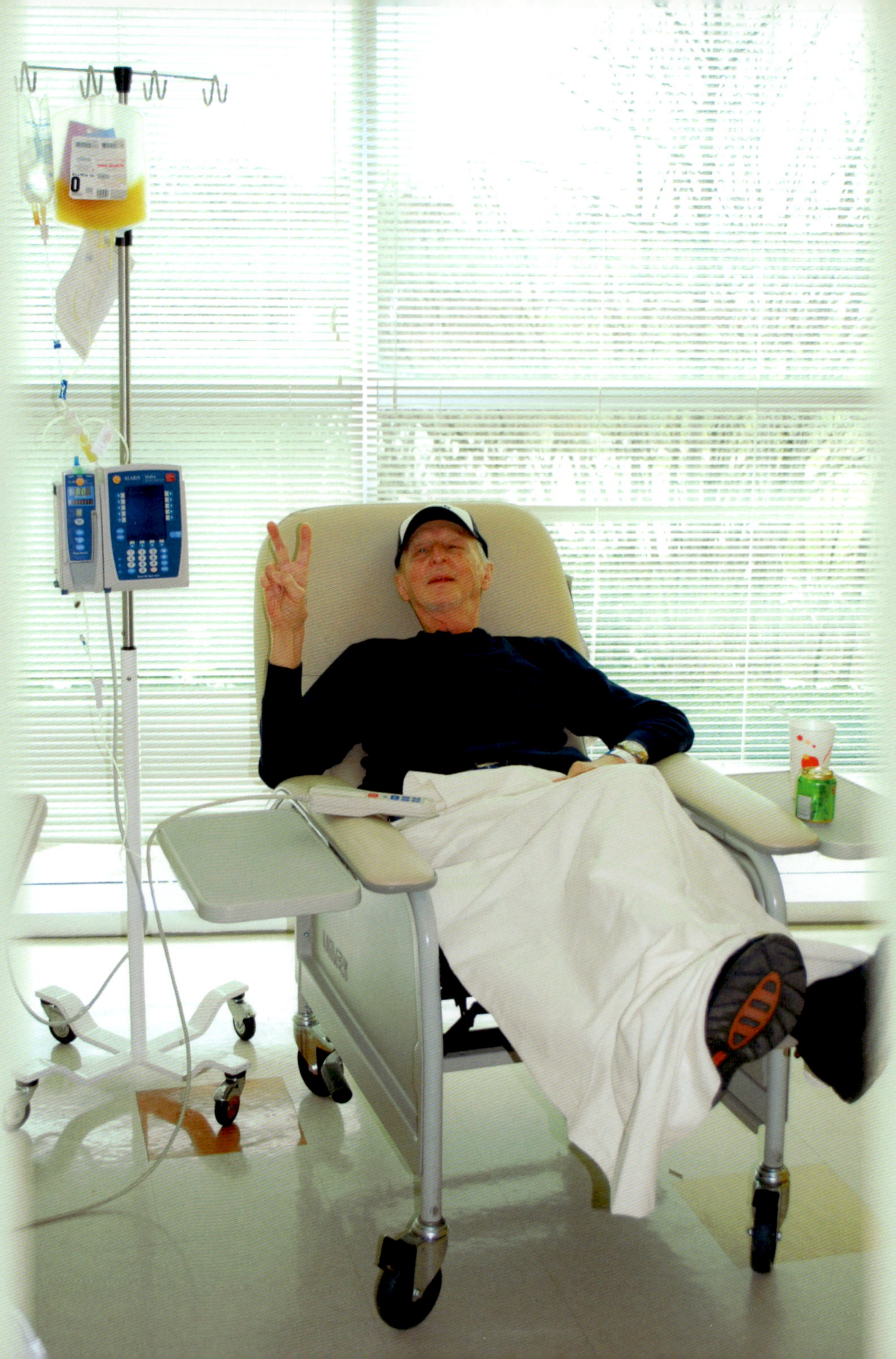

The doctor may want them to have *chemo*.

This is when they put *medicine* in the body.

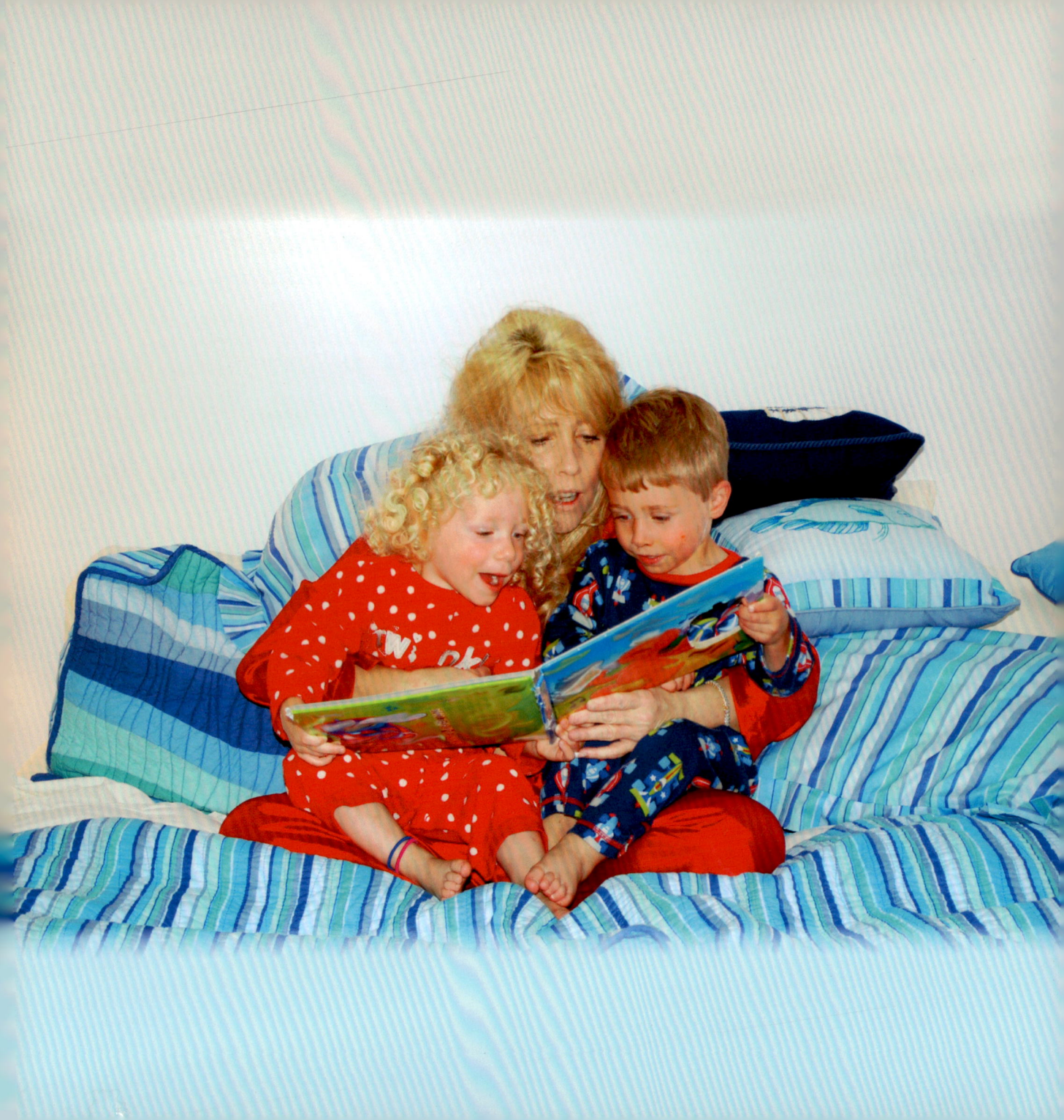

Sometimes after getting chemo they are really tired and sometimes sick . . .

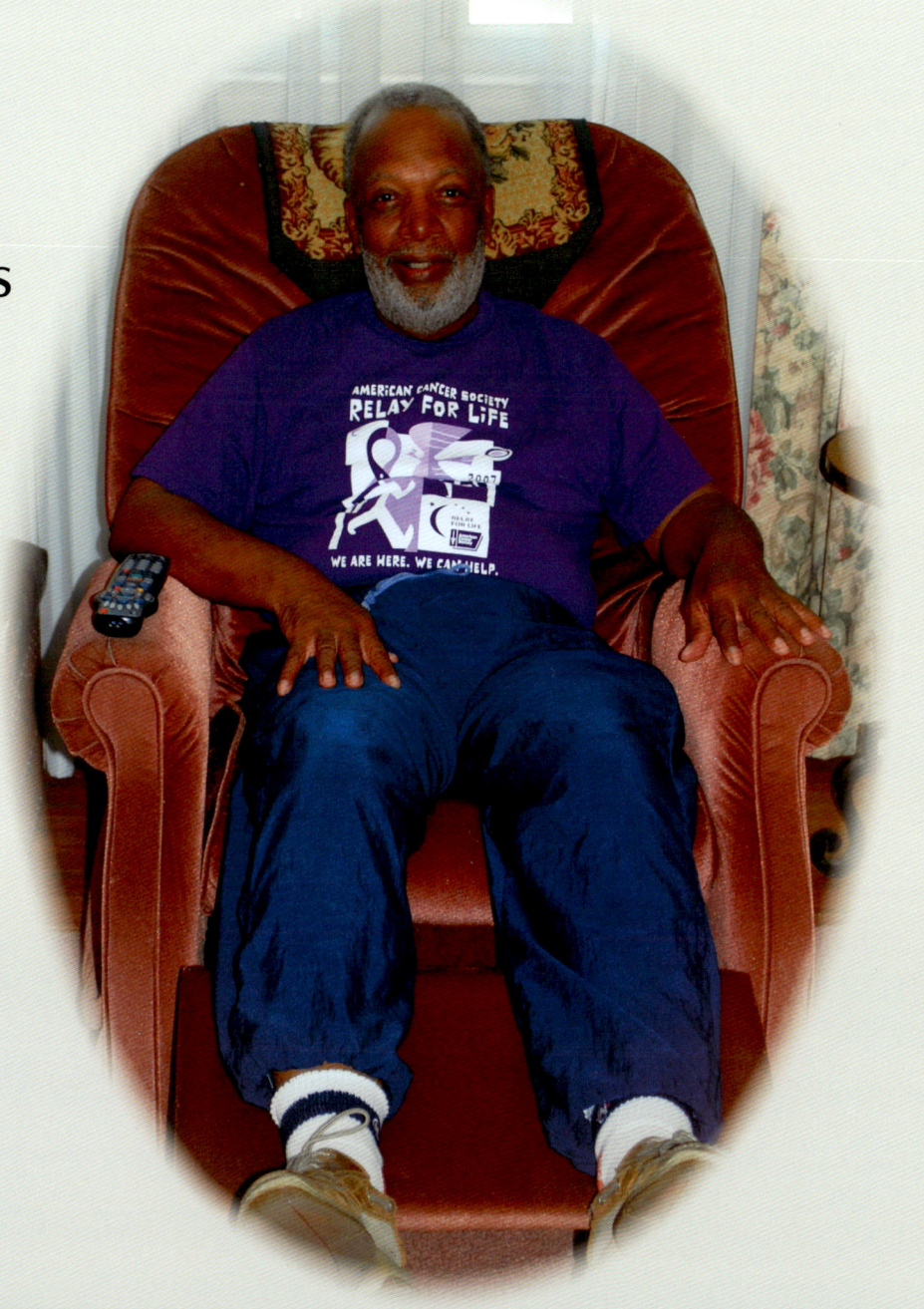

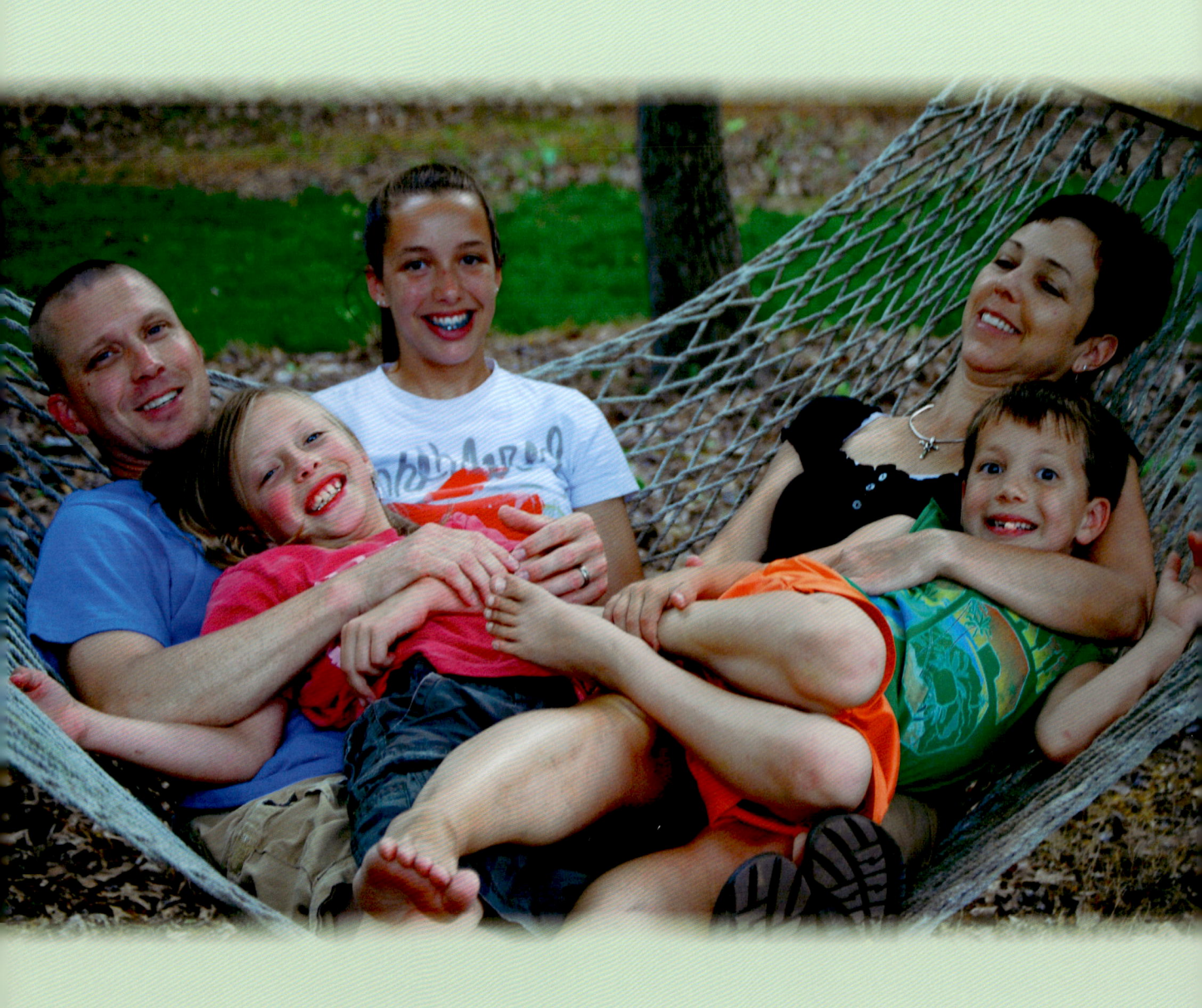

They will need to

get lots of

rest . . .

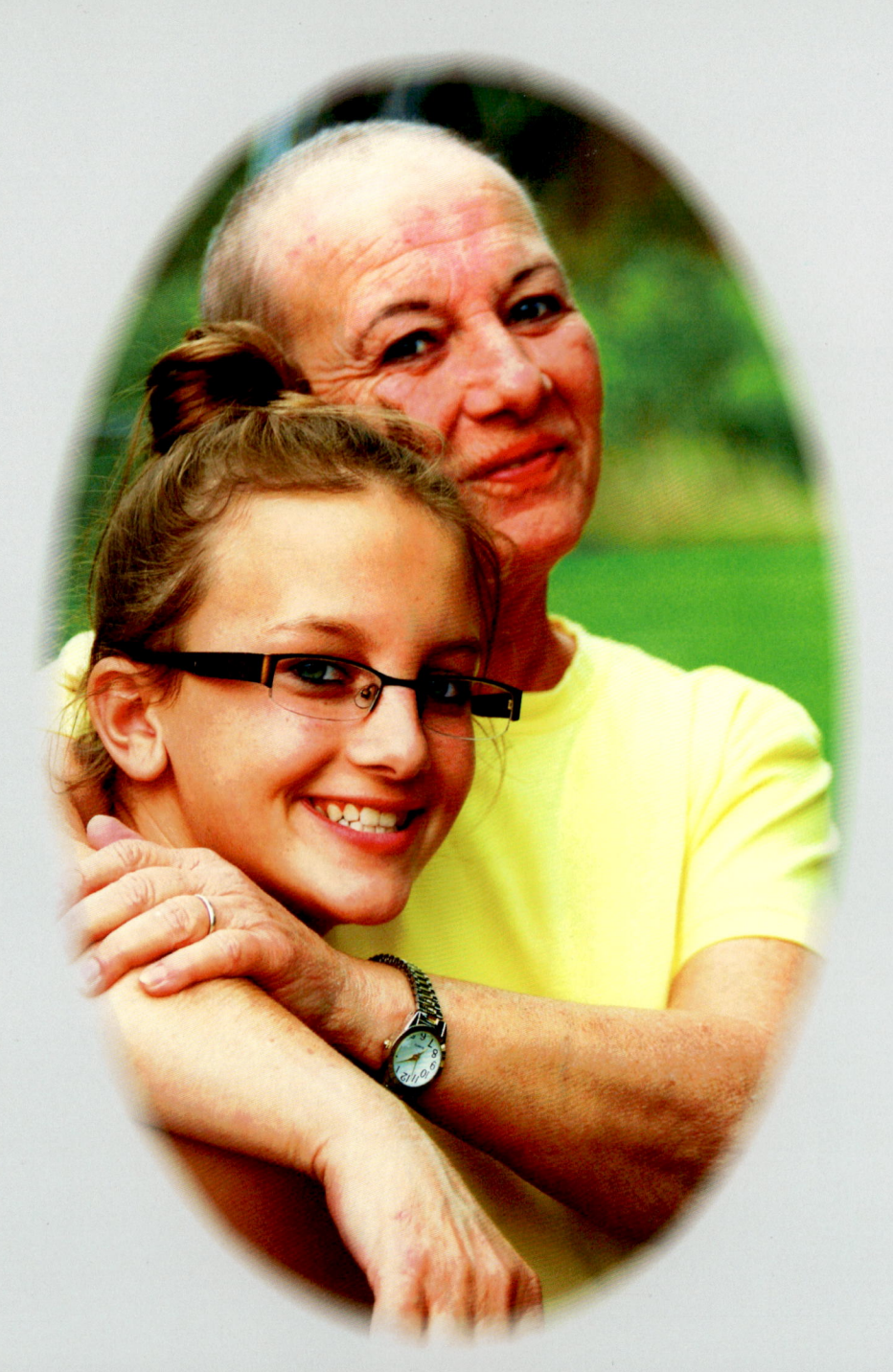

sometimes after
chemo . . .

the medicine will make their hair fall out.

This lets us know the medicine is working.

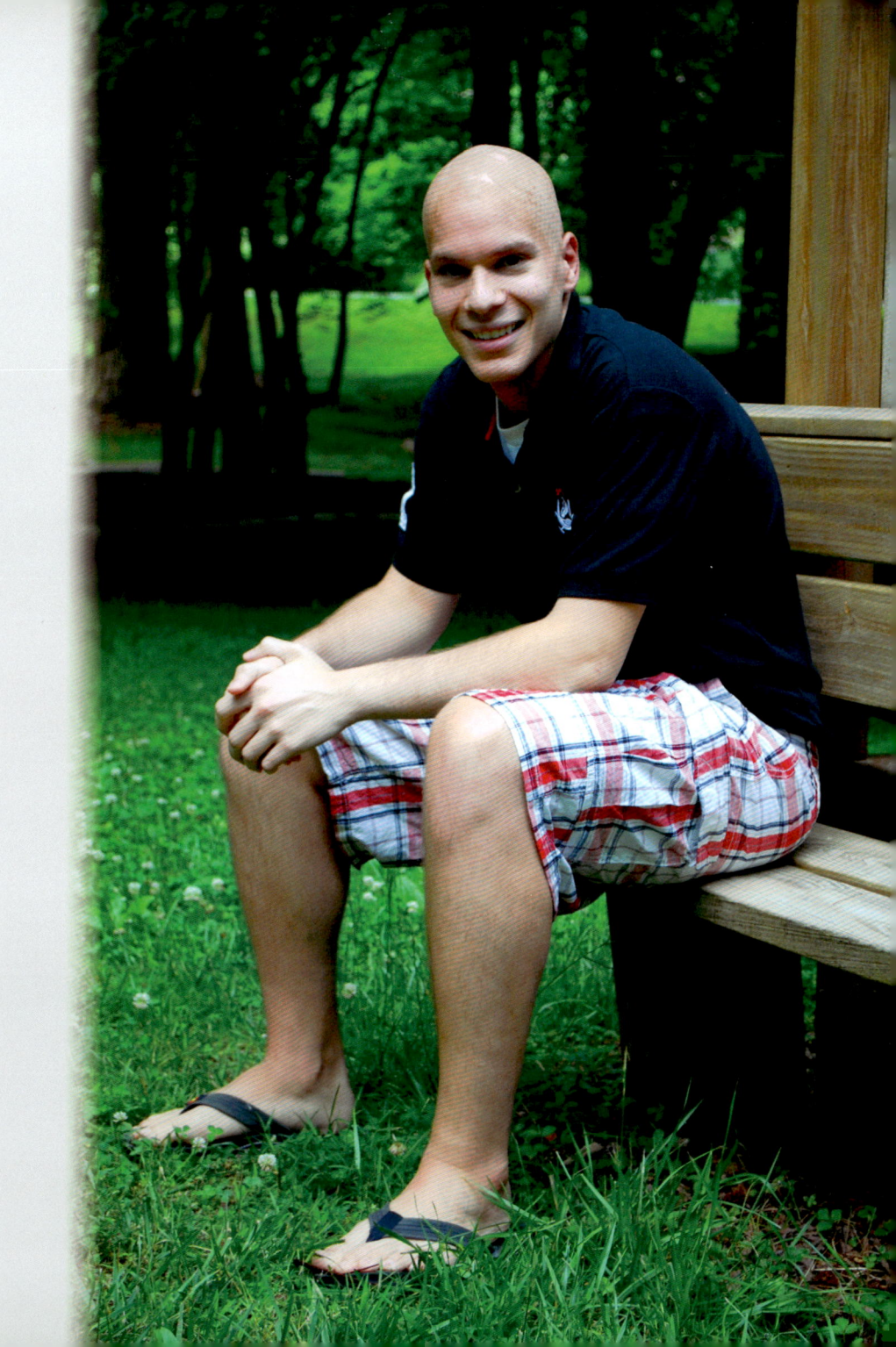

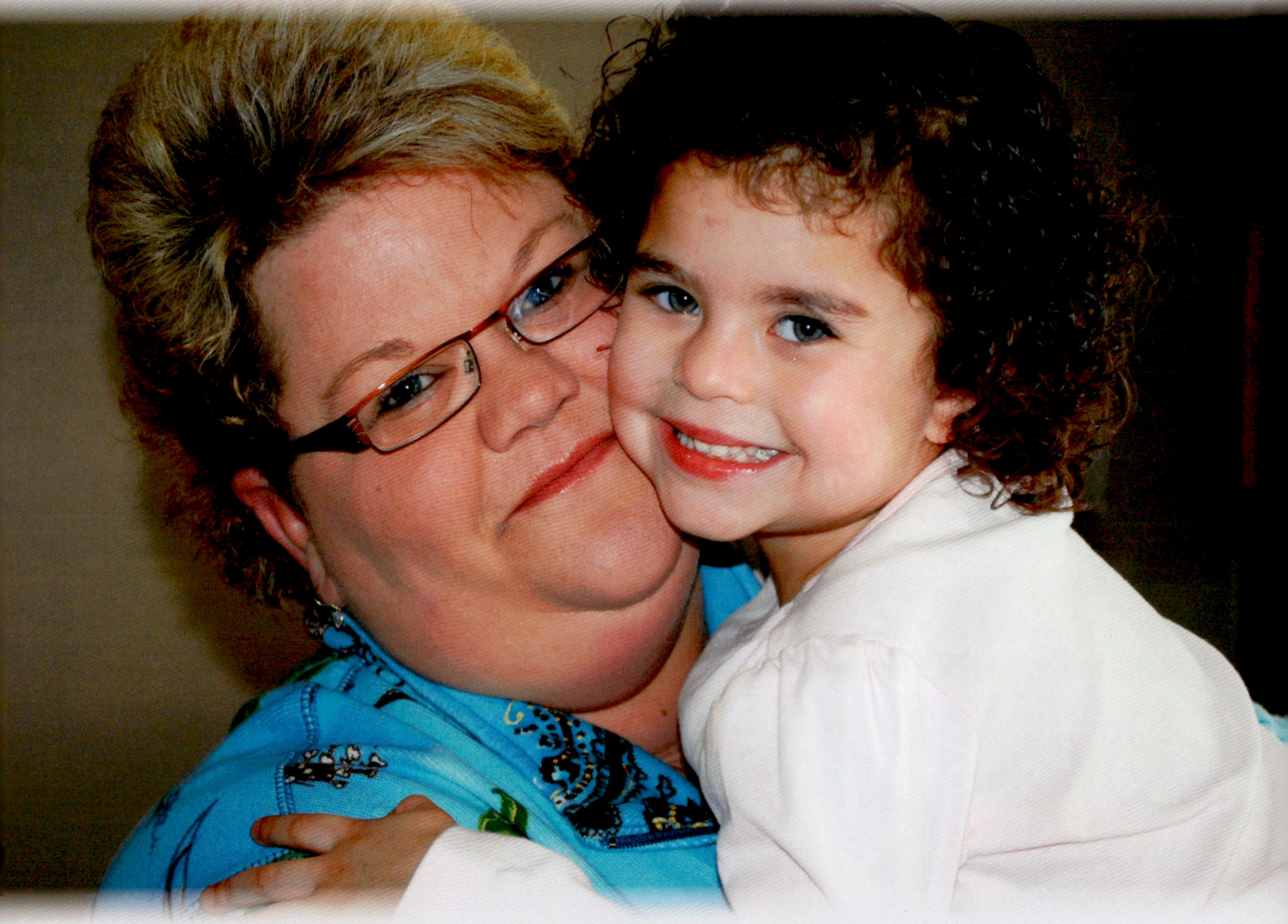

It is very important to let them know you care about them by giving them lots of hugs . . .

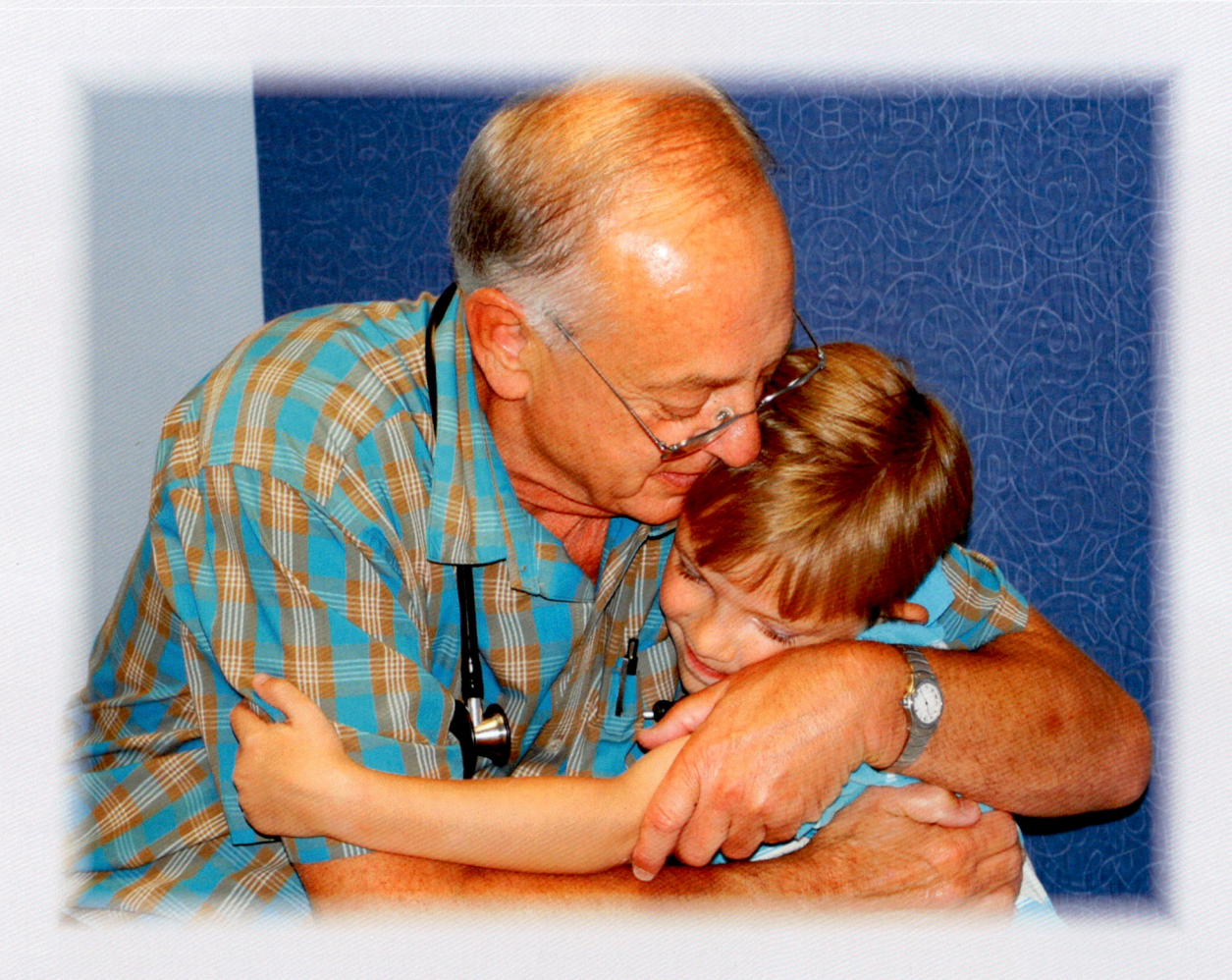

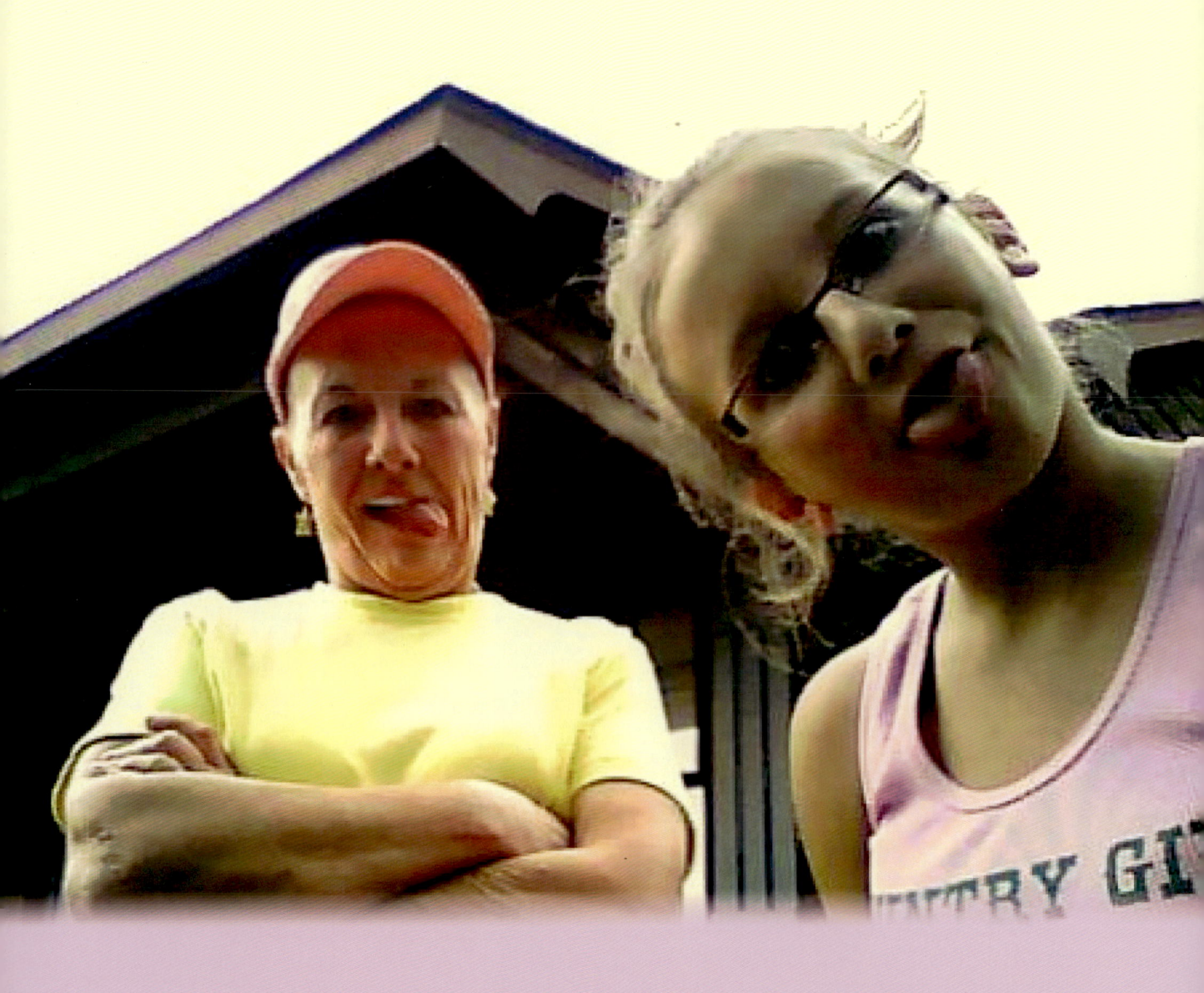

Doctors still don't know how to *cure* cancer; however . . .

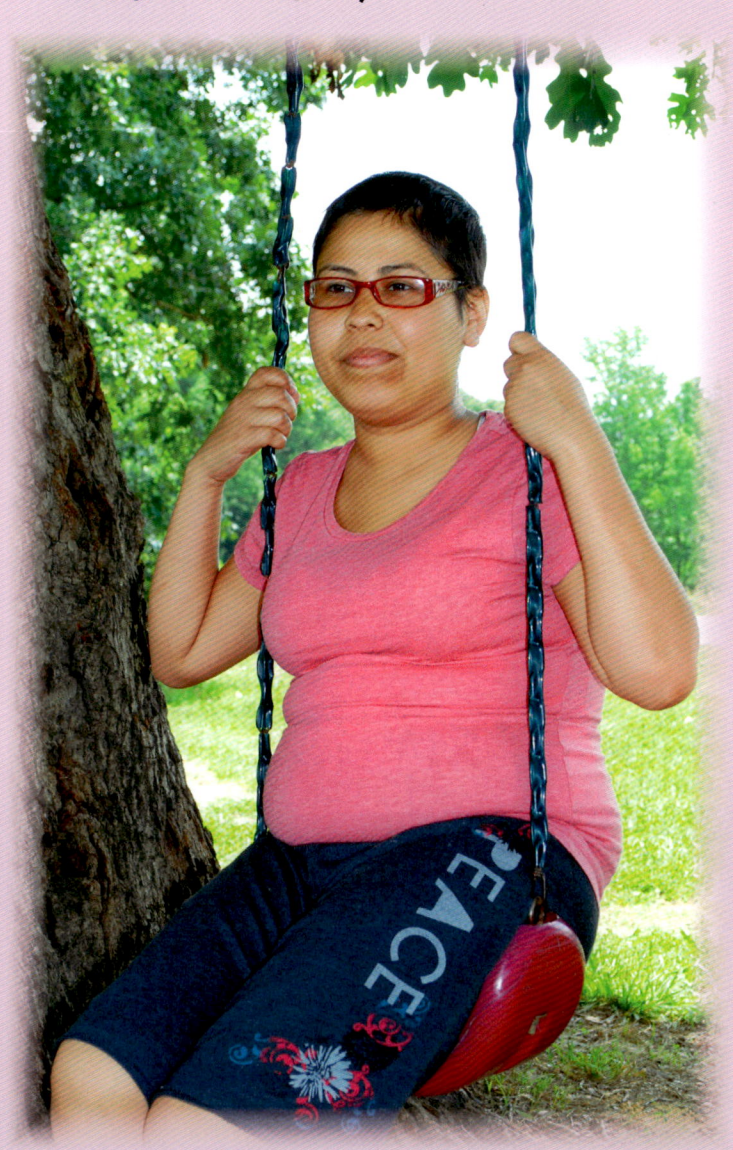

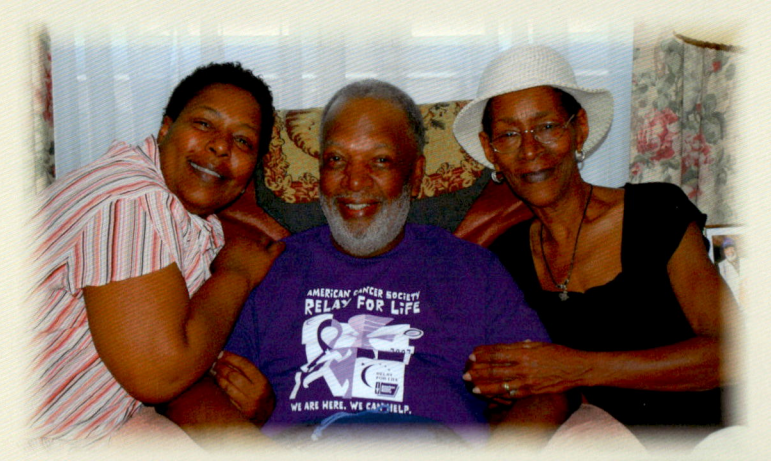

just remember, when someone you love has cancer . . .

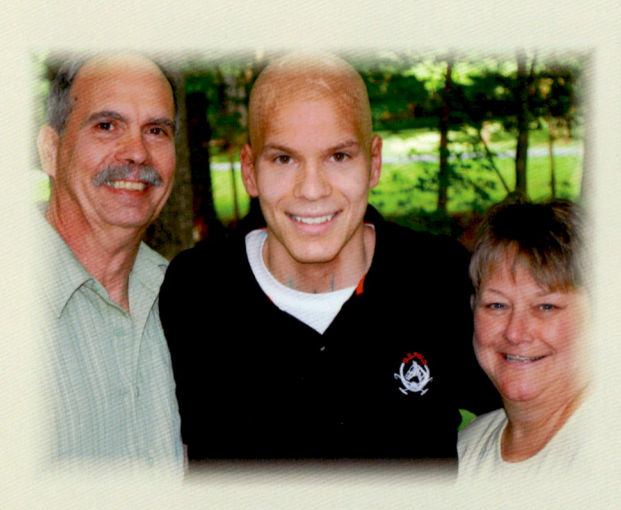

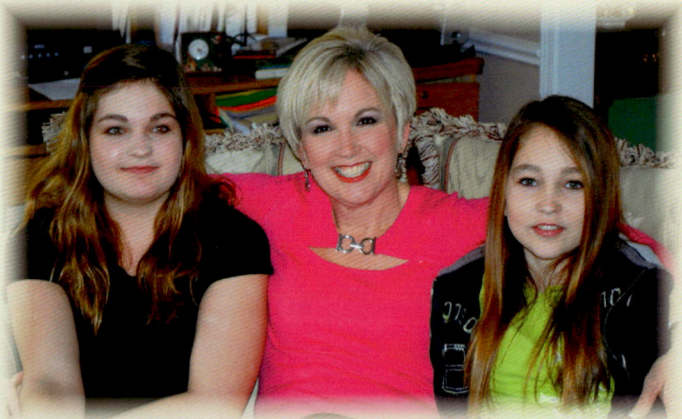

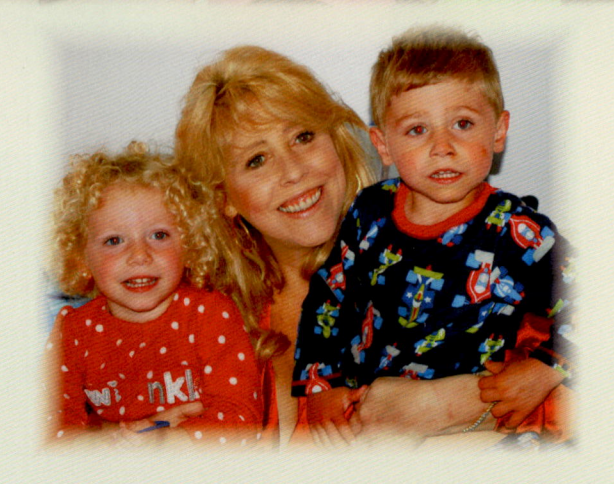

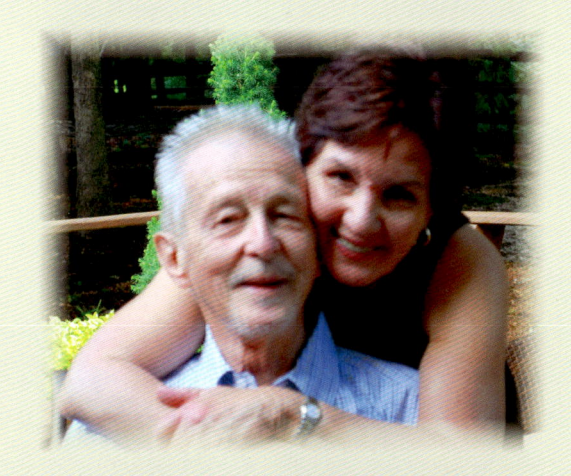

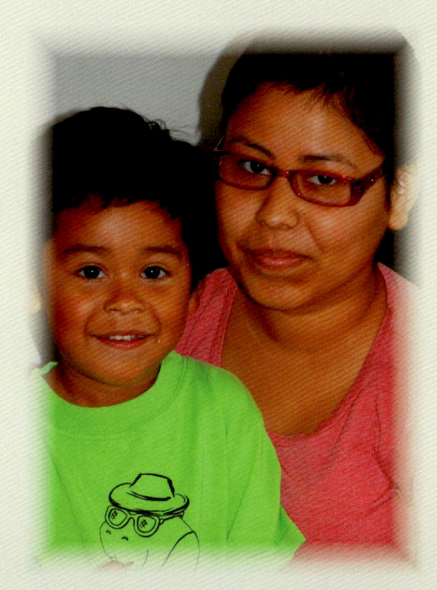

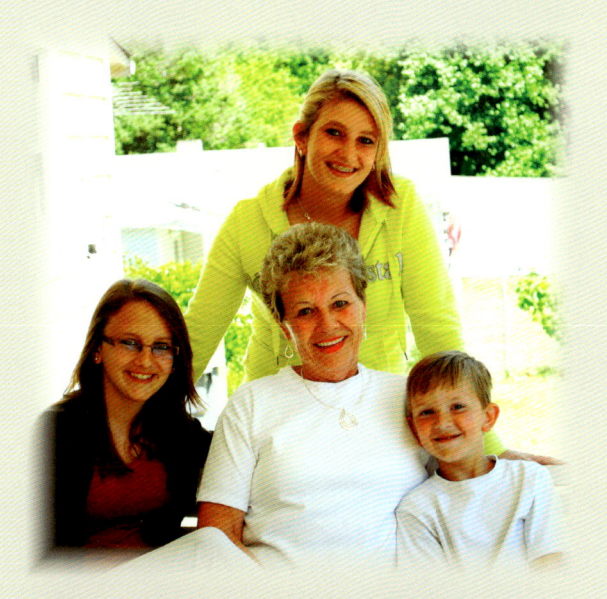

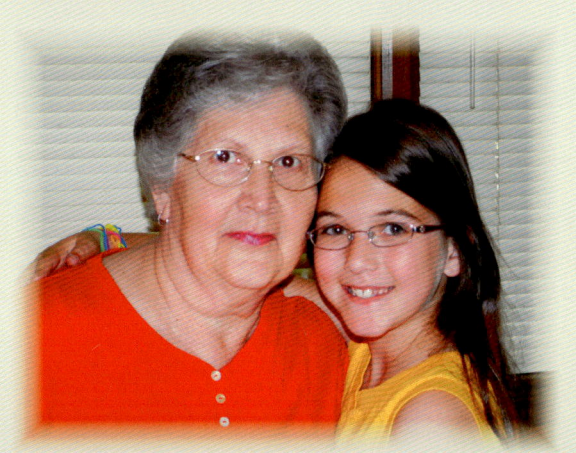

The best thing you can do is let them know how much

You Love Them.

In Honor of:

Louise Bowman
By: Family & Daycare Staff

Cole Chrisley
By: The Jurney Family

Edward Jordan, Jr.
By: Diane & Joe Lewis

Denise Huffman
By: Your Friends at The Children's House

Leigh Nichols
By: Todd, Killian & Rhiannon

Frank Smith
By: Children & Grandchildren

Mary Lee Smith
By: Joseph & Mary Yarborough

Gail Tindall
By: Ray, Alyssa & Katie

Colen Craven
By: Bertha, Children & Grandchildren

Linda Caudle
By: Phil, Tonya & Kids

Vickie Flinchum
By: Gene, Wendi, Dawn & Grandchildren

Ronald Lee Jurney
By: Judy – Children, Spouses & Grandchildren

Joe Lewis
By: Diane, Children & Grandchildren

Juana Ramirez
By: Ramirez Family

Lisa Smith
By: Scott, Ashley, Karley & Garrison

Donna Sprinkle
By: Ray & Gail Tindall

Chris Westmoreland
By: Mom & Dad

Cindy Farmer Wood
By: Bill, Kylie & Abby

In Memory of:

Lorena Anderson
By: Chad & Crystal Ferguson & Kids

Sandra Anthony
By: Lori Cummings

Tyne Burlew
By: Ashley LaPradd

Otis Carter
By: Kenneth Carter

Martha Childers
By: Melissa Eller

Ruby Davis
By: Roger, Christi & Sarah

Chris Eller
By: Katie Eller

Marilyn Routh
By: Tonya, Phil & Kids

Tracy Flinchum
By: The Flinchum Family

Warren "Warden" Grubbs
By: Tim "Tinkerbell" Grubbs

Bebie Hartsoe
By: Kenny Hartsoe

Grandma Betty Hodges
By: Krista, John, Ashlyn & Jordan

Ann Holder
By: John, Jamey, Lisa, Robyn & Families

John Hunsucker
By: Florence, Betty & Lib

Annie Louise King
By: Jerry, Deena, Jennifer, Dale & Jonathan

Lawrence Edward Lane
By: Judy L. Jurney

Helen Louise Bailey Layton
By: Dustin, Krista & Kids

Debaroh Ledford
By: Nicole Moore

Bruce Matweeff
By: Lori Matweeff

Doug McAllister
By: Gwen, Gail, and Doug Jr.

Vera Chavis McCall
By: Isabell Chavis Hawkins

Michael Paszkowski
By: Diane Riley

Lonnie Revels
By: Ruth Revels

Carolyn Sue Riley
By: Cecil Riley

Gary Wayne Simmons
By: Suzie & Chrissie

Wade Spencer
By: Florence

Dick Sprinkle
By: Ray & Gail Tindall

Marshall Tindall
By: Ray & Gail Tindall

Greg Underwood
By: Lori Cummings and Jodi Osborne

Jospehine Yarborough
By: Joseph Yarborough

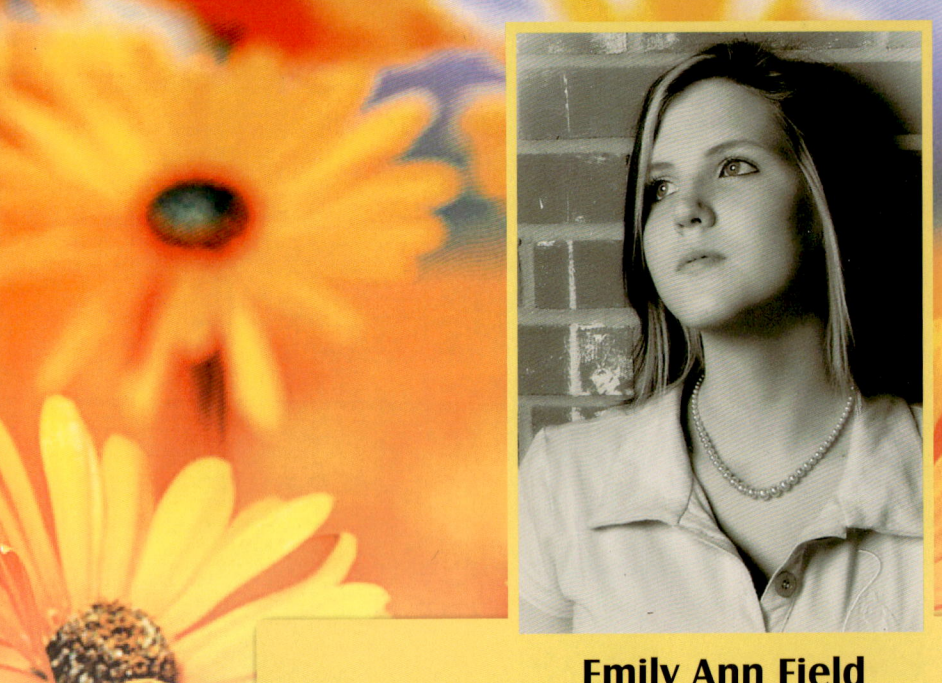

Emily Ann Field
March 31, 1990 – November 22, 2008

Emily's Kids Foundation is a 501c3 established in May 2009,
to help families who are dealing with Pediatric Cancer.
The foundation provides gas cards, parking and meal vouchers for families while they are undergoing treatment.
The foundation is completely dependent on
grants, donations and gifts from businesses and people just like you.

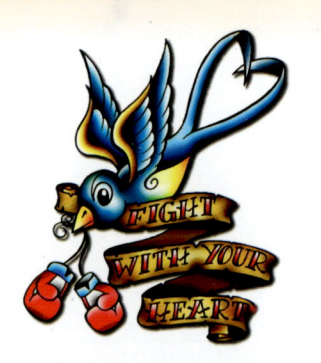

For all of us who have lost someone,
may we always remember their
Strength, their Courage, and their Dignity.

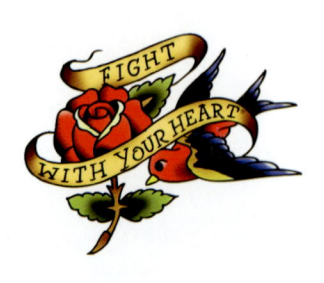

www.emilyskidsfoundation.org